Learning Disability – A Social Approach

The detailed study of learning disability features rarely in university courses. To a large extent this reflects the low value attributed by our society and its human services to people with learning difficulties. This unusual book, based on one of those rare courses, includes contributions from academic specialists, students and people with learning difficulties, all of whom have participated in the course. Its 'social approach' challenges the very idea of what should be taught about the subject of learning disability and who should teach it.

Learning Disability – A Social Approach looks at how people's lives are affected by human services. It covers specific policy and service issues, different aspects of working with people and key debates. The unique insights gained from the combination of academic knowledge and real-life experience make it a topical and thought-provoking text for anyone involved with learning disability – student, teacher, professional or policy maker.

David Race has worked in the field of learning disability for many years in various countries as a researcher, consultant, writer and teacher. He is currently Lecturer in the School of Community, Health Sciences and Social Care, University of Salford, where he is joint programme leader of the MA in Learning Disability Studies.

Learning Disability –
A Social Approach

Edited by David G. Race

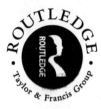

London and New York

First published 2002
by Routledge
11 New Fetter Lane, London EC4P 4EE

Simultaneously published in the USA and Canada
by Routledge
29 West 35th Street, New York, NY 10001

Routledge is an imprint of the Taylor & Francis Group

Typeset in Times New Roman by
Keystroke, Jacaranda Lodge, Wolverhampton
Printed and bound in Great Britain by
St Edmundsbury Press, Bury St Edmunds, Suffolk

British Library Cataloguing in Publication Data
A catalogue record for this book is available from the British Library

Library of Congress Cataloging in Publication Data
A catalog record has been requested

ISBN 0–415–25037–4 (hbk)
ISBN 0–415–25038–2 (pbk)

Contents

Contributors

Kathy Boxall is a freelance consultant and trainer. At the time of writing she was a lecturer in the Department of Applied Health and Social Studies at Stockport College. Her background is in work with children and adults with learning difficulties in education, social services and voluntary sector settings. She also has experience as a volunteer advocate.

Iain Carson is a lecturer in learning disability studies in the Faculty of Education, University of Manchester. He is currently the Programme Director of their BA (Hons) Learning Disability Studies programme.

Errol Cocks is Adjunct Professor of Human Services in the School of Occupational Therapy in the Division of Health Sciences at Curtin University of Technology in Western Australia. He has worked in the disability sector since 1970 in Australia and the UK.

Daniel Docherty is a man who has learning difficulties and is a member of Manchester People First. His special interests are in the areas of sexual awareness and inclusion and he works as a trainer in this area.

Michaela Jones (not her real name) is expecting her third baby. She is hoping that she will get the help she needs and it won't be taken away like her other two children were. Michaela is disabled and has learning difficulties but she doesn't want help from Social Services. She hopes she will get the support she needs from someone else.

John Kenworthy is a clinical psychologist, working with young children and families for the past twenty years; he is presently based in Liverpool. John has a powerful commitment to inclusive education and provides advocate support for families and children who have to struggle for their place within mainstream schools. John challenges conventional thinking related to learning difficulties where it is focused upon the individual and is active in working to make support structures effective and meaningful.

David Race has worked in the field of learning disability for many years in various countries, as a researcher, consultant, writer and teacher. He is currently lecturer in the School of Community, Health Sciences and Social Care, University of Salford.

Sarah Rooney is a lecturer in the Department of Applied Health and Social Studies at Stockport College. She has a background of working with children and young people with learning difficulties in the areas of education and family support. She particularly wishes to acknowledge the valuable contributions to her chapters made by the Norman family and the 'What about the Workers' group in Oldham.

Shaun Smith (not his real name) is a disabled person. He and his partner are expecting their third baby. Shaun attended a Partners in Policymaking course about disabled rights and he has an assignment to do for this. He is also trying to write his life story. Shaun needs help with reading and writing but at the moment he has nobody to help him. Shaun feels there should be more long-term support available for people with learning difficulties who want help with reading and writing.

Joe Whittaker has been a teacher for the past twenty-four years, working in all sectors of education. Joe is presently working in teacher education at Bolton Institute, where he encourages teachers to create learning environments that welcome all learners. Joe has been actively involved in the campaign for inclusive education for many years and argues that segregated schooling is a denial of a person's right to belong, which is damaging to the individual and ultimately the wider community.

Paul Williams has worked in the field of learning difficulties for almost forty years, in residential care, research, staff training and service evaluation. He is currently a lecturer in social work at the University of Reading and was external assessor to the Stockport course in learning difficulties from 1997 to 2001. He is author of a book on self-advocacy by people with learning difficulties and is a management committee member of Citizen Advocacy Information and Training.

Foreword and acknowledgements

Such are the changes and chances of academic life, the world of learning disability services, and, it seems, our very existence, that both the shape of this book and not a few of its authors have been subject to upheavals, revisions and even traumas during its development.

All the more reason, therefore, for me to thank those authors for their efforts. As I outline in the Introduction below, the basic academic task of writing a textbook, which had, until this book, been a relatively straightforward one, had a new dimension, and a creative tension added to it in our attempts to represent the ethos of the degree course at Stockport College with which we were nearly all in some capacity associated. The fact that changes of jobs (and even countries), car crashes, illnesses, and delayed Government White Papers were to come along in the course of the writing only increases those thanks, given what I believe to be the unique quality of the end result.

That, of course, is for others to judge, and we collectively put the contents that follow before them. None of this would have even been possible as a basic idea, however, without the framework of the Stockport course on which to build this book. That framework, as well as involving the contributors to this book, included others not mentioned in the chapters which follow. We do note later the contribution of students and people with learning difficulties to many of the chapters, and as editor I wish to acknowledge that again here, but of the others who taught on the course, individual mention should be made.

Christine McKenna, with her customary intellectual toughness and political acumen, successfully steered the course from a diploma to a degree, through the Scylla and Charybdis of two academic bureaucracies. Then, as director, she began the process of development that was to lead to the high point of creative energy represented by this book. Others who taught on the course but now, like many of us, have gone on different paths, also made their unique contribution to this process. Barbara Brooks, Alan Phipps, Ruth Ridgard and Martin Routledge all need to be acknowledged in this regard. We hope the book is worthy of them.

Finally, I would like to thank Michelle Bacca and Edwina Welham of Routledge for their patience with our various vicissitudes, and the wisdom to see which were, and which were not, beyond our control. Also my current employer, Salford

University, and especially the Associate Head (Research) of my school, Alys Young, for negotiating the space and time for me to edit the book and write my own contributions, amidst the rapid expansion of that school, with its concomitant demands on academic staff time. Though, in the peculiar world of academic research assessment, the book may count no more than a ten-page article in a refereed journal, it is one of the pieces of my work on which I would most like to be judged, and of which I am most proud.

D.G. Race, August 2001

Introduction

David Race

This book is intended to serve two purposes. As it was being written, however, a notion, already apparent but unframed, became clearer. This is that a tension exists between the two purposes, and it is a tension that goes to the heart of the title – *A Social Approach*.

The two purposes were as follows: first, to provide a textbook on learning disability suitable for use in undergraduate and other courses, especially the sort of degree course with which many of the authors of this book were connected, namely what was called the BA (Hons) Professional Studies: Learning Difficulties at Stockport College of Further and Higher Education. In this regard, similarities were drawn with earlier texts with which I have been associated, either as co-author or contributor (Malin *et al*. 1980; Malin (ed) 1995), and initial frameworks followed their structure.

The second purpose, which grew stronger as the book developed, was to try and convey to the reader some sense of the creative energy of that degree course, which I believe was the direct result of an evolving approach to the subject, fuelled by the involvement and interaction of ourselves as staff, the students that we taught, and especially people with learning difficulties with whom we and the students worked. That energy, assisted by supportive external examiners, some of whom have also contributed to the book, resulted, for a relatively brief period of time, in what I can only describe, in the O'Briens'(2000) phrase, as a 'community of practice' approach to the teaching of a degree.

Hence the tension. As will become readily apparent to readers who venture further into the book, an approach to teaching which seeks to involve not only students, but those people who, to all intents and purposes, are the 'subjects of study', in teasing out valuing and respectful ways of working with people with learning difficulties, especially at degree level, is setting itself against a number of conventional wisdoms. These include the hierarchical nature of how knowledge, and access to it, is granted to people in our society, and how those deigned fit to pass on that knowledge are similarly graded. In addition, the notion of what constitutes an 'academically acceptable' textbook is brought into question, and along with it the current government's notions of 'evidence' on which policy decisions might be made.

Though many innovative approaches to teaching and learning were developing in universities and elsewhere, a fledgling degree, developed from a diploma in 1992, taught at a college and externally validated, might have been expected to 'toe the line' of academic conservatism (especially in the post-Thatcher educational marketplace). Instead, reflection on the issues affecting the lives of people with learning difficulties, and the coming together of a stable course team with strong (though not identical) views on which of those issues were important, meant that, gradually, the course developed into an attempt to reflect an approach to learning disability that was distinct from many others.

In addition, however, as two of us noted publicly in early 1999 (Boxall and Race), the course at Stockport was, at that point, the only undergraduate degree course solely concerned with learning disability that did not have nurse training as a principal component. This was not, however, a single-edged sword. As again will be apparent to readers of the rest of the book, people with learning difficulties, and services for them, have tended to be among the least regarded when it comes to the possible attentions of undergraduates, reflecting a similar lack of attention in the population as a whole. To be a unique non-nursing course on this subject therefore had the advantages of innovation but the disadvantages of isolation.

What do we mean, then, by a 'social approach' and why should it cause tension in the writing of a textbook. One answer to this question would be to invite the reader to read the rest of the book, possibly avoiding the tendency in much, even academic, discourse to reduce complex issues to soundbites and slogans. This I do, but to set the reader on their way I will try and relate a few of the emerging issues that coalesce around the notion of a 'social approach'. Some of these are value positions, and as such their wording is my responsibility in writing this introduction, though I would doubt if my colleagues would differ from their essence.

- First, and most important, is the notion that people with learning difficulties have, like everyone else, a value for being, not for being something. What society makes of their identity, and what identity it forces on them, is revealed in many parts of this book, but our starting point is the people themselves, and what this value position states is their inherent worth.
- Second, a degree course, and textbook flowing from that course, if it is to reflect the values position above, must use not just the standard academic tools of textbooks and lectures, but also the views and experiences of people with learning difficulties, and encourage students to reflect on their attitudes and values as much as on their acquisition of 'knowledge'.
- Third, as a result of our own reflection, with no claims for uniqueness or perfection in such results, we conclude that the overall power that guides attitudes to, services for, and much academic teaching about learning disability is how people are perceived by the wider society, and this perception is still largely a negative one. Hence our teaching and our writing, should reflect and challenge this reality, and a course which looks to address the fact of devaluation can best do so by addressing the same forces in society – hence a 'social approach'.

So in the end we have attempted to use the tension creatively, and the structure and language of the book reflects this. We start, in Part I, with a chapter that tries to get a sense of the interactive processes that took place as the degree course developed, focusing specifically on the contributions of people with learning difficulties and our students to those processes. Then, in Part II, much more detail of the context of learning disability services is given, starting with a historical perspective, then addressing various aspects of life which services affect. Residential and day services, education services, and employment services are all dealt with, with critical comment being made by the authors, as well as views on the likely impact of the Government's recent White Paper, *Valuing People: A New Strategy for Learning Disability for the 21st Century* (DoH 2001). Such comment continues in the last two chapters of Part II, where first the organisational and financial impacts are considered, followed by a look at issues of quality in services.

Part III gives three examples of specific issues in working with people with learning difficulties which are among the most closely connected with broader societal attitudes and the response of services. These are: relationships and sexuality; working with people with complex needs; and issues of advocacy, specifically around parents with learning difficulties. In all the chapters of Part III, and two of the chapters of Part II, direct experiences of people with learning difficulties, either in their own words or in true-life accounts, are combined with the results of academic writers to give a picture in keeping with the approach of the course and the book.

In Part IV, two of the more theoretical, but none the less influential issues in academic debate of relevance to learning disability are discussed, namely individual and social models of disability and the so-called 'normalisation debate'. It will be argued that both of these issues have much to offer in aiding reflection on the situation of people with learning difficulties in society.

Finally, in the Conclusion, I attempt to relate broader ethical issues to the findings of the chapters that precede it, with a personal view on the current state of a 'social approach' to learning disability.

Two other matters need to be stated in this introduction. The first concerns the normal caveat that all the authors of chapters in this book are expressing their own views as individuals, and that these do not necessarily represent the views of their present or previous employers. This perhaps needs to be emphasised, because of the references to the course at Stockport. As will be seen from the brief biographical sketches at the beginning, a number of the authors, myself included, taught on the course, whilst others were external examiners, and, as noted above, the book represents, at least to a large extent, the coming together of views on learning disability around that course. Nothing is permanent, however, and the sketches also show that many of us have moved elsewhere. Wherever we are now employed therefore, the views expressed here are our own, with the range of passion and reason that you would expect in any group of individuals.

This leads to the second concluding point, concerning our use of language. As regards the term 'learning disability' one result of a social approach would be, as some have argued in the disability movement, to regard the term itself as either meaningless, or part of societal oppression of disabled people. The first argument follows from the social theory of disability, in that disability – or disablement – is seen as the restriction, discrimination and oppression meted out by society's attitudes and structures towards people with impairments. Therefore 'disabling learning' does not mean anything (except perhaps to describe discriminatory educational practices – see Chapter 4). The second argument sees 'learning disability' as a government imposed label, unique to this country, and therefore adding confusion to international discussion of the issue. This debate itself is worldwide however, and is compounded when some people with learning difficulties say they prefer that term to describe them.

As writers of this book, however, we also want, following the first of the purposes outlined above, for it to be read, and to be recognised as contributing to the area of study with which we are concerned. We therefore have to accept that 'learning disability' is now commonly (and officially) used, at least in the UK, and trying to influence that 'field of study' needs some recognition of the book by those in the field, and those entering the field.

We have therefore adopted a compromise position for the purposes of the book, of using the term 'learning disability' when talking about that 'field of study' or as an administrative classification of services (hence 'learning disability services'), but when talking about people, of using the term learning difficulties (hence 'people with learning difficulties'). We do so, not to confuse, and apologise if we do so, but to reinforce the whole thesis of this book, revealed in language as much as anything else, that the 'social approach' of any given society has power for good or ill over groups it classifies together.

I hope the views of the various authors, some of which were generated over the years of our teaching and interaction with people, will give pause for thought amongst the generation that will be attempting to implement the 'Strategy for the twenty-first century'.

References

Boxall, K. and Race, D.G. (1999) Challenging the medical model, *Community Care,* Inside Supplement, 25 March.

Department of Health (2001) *Valuing People: A New Strategy for Learning Disability for the 21st Century,* London, The Stationery Office.

Lyle O'Brien, C. and O'Brien, J. (2000) *The Origins of Person-Centred Planning: A Community of Practice Perspective,* Georgia, Responsive Systems Associates, Inc.

Malin, N.A. (ed.) (1995) *Services for People with Learning Disabilities,* London, Routledge.

Malin, N.A., Race, D.G. and Jones, G. (1980) *Services for the Mentally Handicapped in The UK,* London, Croom Helm.

Part I

Voices of people

Chapter 1

Attempts at a social approach to a degree course

David Race

Introduction

As the degree course at Stockport progressed in its attempts to become more inclusive, and to give students 'knowledge', not just from the traditional routes of lectures and reading lists, but also by drawing on the lived experiences of people with learning difficulties, a number of innovative ways emerged. This chapter attempts to give a flavour of the results of that innovation, and to start the book with the voices of both students and people with learning difficulties themselves. The chapter is placed first, and as a part in its own right, in recognition of the philosophy within which the course, and gradually the book, developed, as discussed in the Introduction.

The authors are many and varied, and are named where permission has been granted by the individuals concerned. One of the authors of other chapters, Kathy Boxall, was responsible for gathering the various opinions, and is named, as is Iain Carson, the former Course Director, in some of the accounts. With one exception Kathy also wrote the introductory remarks. The Editor was responsible for the order and format of the chapter as a whole. Each piece will be set in context, but the broad aspects of the course that are covered are: people with learning difficulties as presenters; as participants in research for dissertations; and as providers of criteria by which students on placements, in their role as 'staff', might be judged.

David Barron

Introductory remarks

As a child, David Barron was institutionalised under the 1913 Mental Deficiency Act. He spent many years at Whixley Institution near York and was finally released in the 1950s. Since then, David has written his autobiography *A Price to be Born* (Barron 1996) and has become an accomplished orator, speaking and lecturing to many groups ranging from primary school children to university students.

Since 1992, David has given an Annual Lecture to students on the BA (Hons) Professional Studies: Learning Difficulties at Stockport College. Below is David's view of teaching at Stockport – transcribed from a tape made in his flat on 12 August 2000 (two days after his 75th birthday).

David Barron's view of teaching

I've now stopped lecturing over at the Holy Family school in Leeds where I've been going for the past twenty-two years. I would like to have carried on there, but the headmaster's taken early retirement and so has the organiser who arranges for me to speak to the children. I found that by speaking to those children it was great because, with living in Leeds myself as a child, I was able to give them a bit of local history.

However, coming back on to Stockport College, I've always said out of the countless schools and colleges I've been to and the Open University and the Royal College of Nursing and the church groups, I found the other place, besides the Holy Family school, that I've liked going to most of all is Stockport College. Some places look so nice on the surface but when you get down to it, you're not talked to, they talk down to you. That I didn't like, but I still went and still tried to get my life story across regarding the institution where I was a patient for twenty-five years. I can always tell when I walk into the room what sort of reception I'm going to get. I've always been received very well by both the students and staff alike on the learning difficulties course at Stockport College. There's only one thing that hurts me more than anything, and this I must say.

On one occasion, I did have, from Stockport College, five students come to visit me at my home as they were so impressed with the talk I'd given them about the time I spent at Whixley Institution. They were the only ones that came. After that I only received the occasional Christmas card from the odd student, certain ones. It does hurt me. You go and speak to a class of students like I did just this last year, the year before we came into 2000. I found that the students promised me faithful that they would send me a card and some wanted to come and see me. It was only a small group and they were very, very taken up with everything I was saying, in fact the time went literally so fast that it was over before you knew where you were. At the end of the day I do get upset though because they promised they would come and see me, two students, they promised they would come, but they didn't, none of them. I stop and think these students have a tremendous lot to do, they haven't got the time to visit me.

The thing that helps me is that I know that it's embedded in them, something I've said which is going to help them in their course or in their work and this in turn will help other people. At the end of the day if it's what the students want and the powers that be are prepared to have me in Stockport College, then I'm fully prepared to go. If I can carry on, then I know that when God takes me off this earth, then at least I'll have left a message that in some cases will be able to stop the tremendous cruelty that's taken place, not just to me, but to thousands of patients alike.

Now the other reason for my talking the way I do, and as painful as it is when I am talking on the subject of my life in the institution, is I stop and think of the countless thousands that there must have been in the institutions. I also stop and think of the poor souls in the community today who can't speak out for themselves. In a way, I'm trying to speak out for them.

I lectured for ten years at the Manchester University. One year when I was at the Manchester University it was the students' Christmas party and they even stayed behind to get my address so they could contact me when they could have just have left the building and gone to their party straight away. So that must have proved that they were really interested in what I said.

I find the students at Stockport have listened attentively to what I have to say too. The must do, otherwise they couldn't ask all the questions they do. They have shown a great interest and they've been very quiet during the lectures. There's not been anybody looking at their watches to see when it's going to be half-time or the end. It's always been a case of me saying, 'Have I got any time left?' That's how it's been over and over again with the students at Stockport College.

On my last visit to Stockport College, in the year leading up to the millennium, I was received by a small group of students. I found the students to be very, very impressive right the way through. But what I did, I decided to change a little bit of the way I speak. Instead of leaving it to half-time before giving them a chance to ask questions I gave them the chance to ask questions as I was talking. I said, 'Look, I'll stop if you want to ask me a question now'. I found that it went over better and the students did too. But there again, at the end of the day they asked for my address but I haven't heard from them.

The only thing I was worried about the last time I came to Stockport College was when Iain and Kathy said, 'This is the last time you're coming to the College, isn't it David?'. Well, the bottom nearly dropped out of me because I thought I really don't want to stop coming to Stockport College. Even if they say they can't afford to give me any money at all, I still want to keep going there. As I've said before, the Holy Family school in Leeds and the Stockport College mean more to me than anything else on this earth. Then they said, 'Well we thought that you'd said you wanted to retire David'. I said, 'No, it must have been a misunderstanding because in no way do I want to give the College up until the College decides it wants to get shot of me. Well when they said, 'There's no fear of that David', that lifted me up. So that visit was a tonic and I got a good reception from the students. Two students were going to come to visit me – sadly, that didn't materialise. Another five students were going to write to me. Now in all fairness I may have received a card from one of them. I think it's only that that does hurt me a bit. But they definitely do take notice. You might say well how do you know if they take notice or not, David? Well, the answer is if they're not listening, then how could they ask questions?

I'm looking forward to coming to the College again next year and if this book comes to fruition and I'm still alive I would love to receive a copy.

There's one more thing I'd like to say. I only hope that God spares me long enough whereby I can come to the Stockport College and lecture again next year. That would make it ten years that I've lectured at Stockport College, which would make it the same as I did at Manchester University.

Students' views on David's lecture

David returned to Stockport College on 10 January 2001 to give his tenth Annual Lecture. The following week, students were asked to provide written feedback on the lecture. All of the feedback was positive and emphasised the emotional impact and learning from a 'first-hand' account. Sample comments are included below, from a number of different students.

> The talk was very interesting, highlighting the injustice and lack of vision, with regard to people with learning difficulties, perpetrated by officialdom. It is good to see that out of such negativity and discrimination there has been a positive result. I admire your self-confidence and ability to speak before a group of people.

> It was a good experience to actually hear the truth about what went on in the institutions, instead of reading accounts from book. We had the chance to ask questions which was good. Very moving and emotional to think what people went through.

> It was very moving, compelling and in a sense shocking, to hear a person's account first hand, of their life in an institution. It was very beneficial to us all, both personally and professionally to hear David's story. David was extremely open and honest with us – his lecture was excellent – made me see many things in a completely different perspective.

> David's talk was a moving way to gain insight into long-stay hospitals and what people experienced there. David is a very brave man whom we were lucky enough to meet and be allowed to share his experiences. David gave a very open and factual talk that benefited us all and was a very useful learning experience.

> The talk you gave last Wednesday was riveting and fascinating. You were very brave in everything you went through. I cannot believe that this sort of thing can happen in an institution in which a person is supposed to be looked after by people of authority, and not victimised. More people who have been victimised in the early years and who were put into institutions should speak out and tell others about their experiences – good and bad. I read a couple of pages of your book and found it interesting. David, you are an inspiration to us all.

I think having guest speakers with learning difficulties coming into the College is an essential part of the course, to learn mutual respect. It is a good opportunity to listen and learn from a different, non-biased point of view. We get an insight into the courage and determination of some people who would be labelled as dependent and not worth listening to. I would like to see more teaching staff with learning difficulties coming on to the course.

I felt it was great to hear such an honest and open account of David's life. The lecture was emotional for me, though not through a sense of pity. The insight into this man's life and experiences, told so bravely, highlights how services have advanced and also how they must continue to improve for people with learning disabilities. I thoroughly enjoyed David's lecture and I have thought and spoken of him on numerous occasions already.

Hearing David's story of his life enabled myself to understand what it was like to live in an institution. All too often we only hear professional accounts of the effects of being institutionalised – David's story is the real account and therefore is of more importance.

I found David's story very interesting and informative, which gave me enormous insight to life in an institution. David's story being a personal account of his experiences left a deep impression on me of the horrendous situation people faced in an institution because he shared from a feelings and emotional perspective rather than just a factual viewpoint. I believe David's lecture will leave a lasting impression on me in terms of how I conduct my future work practices.

David talked about his institutional years so matter-of-factly, yet at the same time you could feel the pain of those stolen years. I felt the talk was his 'own therapy' – this being David's podium to express his anger about his years of abuse. It was an interesting and yet sad talk; informative and emotive. David had achieved so much in his lifetime and yet had he ever really left the institution? I felt he had (internally) 'stopped living' and he was in a time warp, constantly reliving his time at Whixley Hospital. David appeared not to have come to terms with his years of abuse and yet at the same time appeared so calm and 'in control'. I felt many emotions during (and after) the talk but the most overwhelming feeling was the damage humans inflict on each other – the repercussions can last a lifetime, and in David's case may do.

David has been fronting lectures for the last ten years and I think I speak for each of the students who have attended these lectures when I say that they were extremely moving, informative and relevant. The way in which he explained the experiences and oppression he went through was sobering and necessary and I greatly thank him for how much he taught me in such a short time.

Shaun Smith and Michaela Jones (names have been changed)

Introductory remarks

Shaun Smith and Michaela Jones first became involved with the course in 1998. Initially they worked with two final-year students, Nicola and Michelle, who helped them with writing a book. Shaun and Michaela knew one of the tutors on the course and asked if she could find someone to help them write a book about what happened to them when Social Services removed their children. They wanted to write their book so that more people would know about what happened to them, so that it would be in the 'public eye'.

Nicola and Michelle were undertaking research in related areas for their final year dissertations. The four of them worked together, sharing resources and information. Shaun and Michaela's comments about working with Nicola and Michelle are below.

Shaun and Michaela's experiences

We wanted to write a book about what happened to us, how we felt when Social Services took our children away. We started a [literacy] course at college, one hour a week on a Thursday, and we weren't very satisfied with it because an hour soon goes by and it wasn't enough time. The problem was the college staff wanted us to use the time to fill in their forms but we wanted to get on with writing our book. We spoke to Kathy about it because she was our advocate. Kathy found two students on the course who wanted to help us write our story. That's how we got to know Nicola and Michelle.

Nicola and Michelle told us their course was about helping disabled people in the community and how to get better rights in life. They helped us write things out for our book, correcting spellings and that and helped us to get on the computers in college, usually for about two hours on a Thursday. We had a laugh; they had good sense of humour! We got on. They couldn't be there all the time but they helped us a lot on the computer. It was a good thing, working with Nicola and Michelle, but there's a lot of work still needs doing on the book editing and altering and that.

Nicola and Michelle helped us with doing research for our book. They went up to Yorkshire with us on the train. After Tony was born, we went to a place in Yorkshire. We wanted to interview the people who used to work there about what they thought about the removal of our children; and about how things could be better in the future, for other parents. We asked the questions and Nicola and Michelle wrote things down.

Shaun and Michaela as lecturers

Shaun and Michaela also wanted to talk to the other students in Nicola and Michelle's group, so that they too would know about what happened to them. In order to do this, Shaun and Michaela were employed as visiting lecturers and were supported to prepare and deliver their lecture. They have continued to speak to other groups of students, the most recent occasion being in January 2001. Their comments about speaking to students on the course are below.

> We felt confident when we spoke to the students. The students were quite alright, they understood. People know it's gone on – children being taken away – but they don't know it's actually gone deeper, you know what I mean? One thing I don't like is when there's proceedings going on, when they go to court, they work together all the time, all the different people what are supposed to be on your side. They go in another room and you stay in the background and you don't know what they're up to. When things happen like this with children, I think it should be more or less in the public eye. You know watching what they're up to, not having meetings all the time behind closed doors. People need to know. That's why we want people to know what happened to us.
>
> The students were paying attention, writing it all down on paper. They listened. But when you have somebody's mobile 'phone going off, it's very distracting when you're talking. I should have said, 'Excuse me when your mobile 'phone goes off, do you mind going outside', instead of waiting 'til the end to say it. It's alright talking about it but we want it to get it further afield, not just talking about it, we want to get action about it.

Students' views on Shaun and Michaela's lecture

The students were asked for written feedback about Shaun and Michaela's recent lecture. All of the comments were positive and the lecture clearly had considerable impact. Sample comments are included below.

> Shaun and Michaela are a very close and loving couple. They gave an honest and open account of their experiences, and their feelings at present. The lecture highlighted the fact that no matter how compliant and honest Shaun and Michaela were with Social Services, they were not met with the same respect. I wish the couple all the best with their future hopes and dreams.

> Shaun and Michaela's story was interesting and informative. You could tell how much Shaun cared about his children and how much he resented the way the Social Services treated him and Michaela. They are both extraordinary people, do not let anybody stand in your way and carry on fighting for what you believe.

It was interesting to hear first hand of the experiences that still happen to parents with learning difficulties. It is a sad indictment of society's prejudice that this attitude still exists in the 21st century.

I found your story upsetting and disturbing and unbelievable that this can happen, however I'm not too surprised at the actions of Social Services, knowing and having experienced how they operate. Thanks for sharing your story. Good luck with your work and your book.

Shaun and Michaela – very good to hear their point of view of what happened to them. Showed us all the need for more independent support and advocacy services (free independent support and advice). Makes me want to find out more about the legal rights of people with learning difficulties. Shaun and Michaela were not involved in decision making at all. The way they have been treated is against the Human Rights Act. Where can they turn? They have been blatantly discriminated against. They seriously need an independent advocate to help them get direct payments so they can live life without being summoned and controlled by Social Services.

I found their story very helpful, but also unbelievable. I think it's very sad that this country does not support new families and separates people/families for no valid reason. It is very upsetting and it has made me more determined to provide support for individual people who have a disability. I wish you both all the best for your future and hope everything works out. You can see just by looking at you the love you both have. Your story was very interesting and made me realise how important it is for me to work with people with learning difficulties and not for Social Services. Take care.

Your story was very moving. I feel disgusted that you were treated as you were. I have great respect for the both of you. Thank you for allowing me to have an insight into your lives.

Shaun and Michaela gave a moving example of how unjust our country is and the inequality that people with learning difficulties encounter. Shaun and Michaela are bloody fantastic!!! Our country should be deeply ashamed! I can't believe that our society can let this happen to people. This issue needs airing in public because I believe that many other people would not support this in society as it is today. I am disgusted.

Thanks for coming to talk to us. Your story is very moving, you are brave individuals and it must be so frustrating. I cannot imagine how hard this must have been for both of you. Thanks for sharing this story with us.

Dear Shaun and Michaela. Thank you so much for coming. It takes great strength of character to present your tragic story to us, and I hope the knowledge you have shared with us will help us to challenge the system if we ever find ourselves in the same situation. Thank you again.

Kevin Chettle – Advocacy in Action

Introductory remarks

An organisation that regularly sent speakers to the course was a Nottingham-based group called 'Advocacy in Action'. This group is made up of service users from different backgrounds, including people with learning difficulties. Speakers are provided for various courses, including national and international conferences. Kevin Chettle responded to our invitation to talk about user-led teaching in his own words, including a plug for his home-based university and course, which, as you will hear, he is involved with at a number of levels.

Kevin Chettle in his own words on the value of user-led teaching

I'm an interesting well-known person and I mix with all sorts of people. I'm a famous artist and proud to have been on television. My life is better than the one before – which was terrible when I spent a long time in a hospital locked away from society. It's good now to have a future to look forward to – instead of being kept down and out all the time.

I've been around the country teaching – and abroad for the first time as well – speaking at different conferences and doing all sorts of training events. I've been to so many different universities – I like it – it's good – learning the social workers all about people like me.

And at Nottingham University – I was part of the original planning group that helped to build up the plan about what the Diploma in Social Work Course should be about and how the students could learn all about their values and their knowledge and their skills. I was very proud that this part of the course got a Top Class Mark from the Social Service Inspectors when Nottingham University was inspected.

I feel I'm an important teacher because the students need to hear my point of view instead of making all their assumptions about what I can't do in life and what my 'special needs' are – because I'm the one that's got the experience and I'm the one that's living my life.

And I wish for the students to be confident and challenge all the systems. I wish – when they move into their top jobs – that they listen – really listen – to the people they serve – and work with them together – respecting the people – in equal quality partnerships.

Experiences of working together to complete a dissertation – Nicky Bentley and 'the group'

Introductory remarks – Nicky Bentley

I graduated from Manchester University in July 1999, having successfully completed my degree – BA (Hons) Professional Studies: Learning Difficulties at Stockport College. Throughout my attendance on the course I worked part time supporting eleven adults who had learning difficulties, within their home. The people I supported were a great influence on my studies from the very beginning as their lives truly reflected the subject of many of my lectures. They were in the best position to advise and guide me in both my working practice and my studies.

It was a natural progression, therefore, that in year three of the degree my research project (dissertation) be carried out with the people who had lived the experiences I was hoping to discuss. For the best part of a year I worked with four of the residents of the house where I worked, and together we produced a piece of research entitled: 'Moving House – From An Institution Into The Community'. Nearly two years after the completion of our project we came together to discuss our experiences of carrying out such an intense piece of work together. Only three of the original four group members were able to participate, as one person (Rose) had moved back to live at the institution. Prior to beginning our discussions we talked about how to record this, and the subject of anonymity. The group decided to remain anonymous and are referred to as 'the group'. The place where they used to live is referred to as 'the institution' .

Very simply, I (Nicky) have noted the comments made by the group as we were talking. The group members chose the areas for discussion.

Doing the project with someone we knew well

* You knew something about our background – what we had been through.
* Made it easier to talk – open up.
* Didn't know how they (someone unknown) would react to what we said.
* They might have told the bosses at the institution.
* Wouldn't have trusted them – couldn't have been honest.
* Might have lied.

Being able to talk about our achievements

* Felt good. Realised how much more we do now.
* Meeting people, going out – different places – we never did that at the institution.
* Talking – it was good.
* I know now we were wrapped up in cotton wool – surrounded by the same faces seven days a week. You start to think it's OK when you are there – it's not.

- I know I can do a lot now.
- I needed a hand that's all. Just like the poem said.
- Oh yes, the poem. It made me feel good. Not sad. I'm glad I said yes when they asked me if I wanted to move.
- We are living proof that living in the community is far better. Looking at us as real people – not objects.
- Still want to do more – but it's good to talk about things from the past.

Summary

From the group

Revisiting our project was excellent. We were ready to talk about it once again, to think about the work that we carried out together and to talk about how we are feeling now. Just having some time to reflect felt good.

From Nicky

It never ceases to amaze me how the individual group members have the ability to talk openly about difficult situations and feelings, and then to learn from it and move on. Most of the time, having a laugh about it along the way. Working with the group taught me so much, and although I no longer work with them in their home, I often visit so that they continue to guide me in my work now.

Outside experts – Advocacy in Action

Guidelines for staff

In 1996, with a view to better reflecting the range and diversity of placement and employment opportunities in the learning disability field, it was decided to review the Level Two placement on the BA (Hons) Professional Studies: Learning Difficulties. Part of this process of review involved meeting with placement providers and employers and inviting their comments and feedback. A similar process was undertaken with service users. Ideally these service users would all have had experience of working with students from the course. In practice, they were a group of twelve students with learning difficulties who attended a local college.

Between them, this group had experience of a range of settings including Further/Adult Education classes, Local Authority Day Centres, Local Authority hostels and group homes, voluntary sector residential provision, supported tenancies, NHS group homes and (historically) hospital/institutional provision. None of them, however, had direct experience of working with a student on placement from the course.

The group was approached and asked to help with the review. They were keen to participate and were asked what they thought students needed to know before they went on placement. This was a difficult concept for people to grasp. It became apparent, as the discussion progressed, that it wasn't easy for some people to differentiate between students, staff, volunteers etc. It also became clear that the distinction wasn't necessarily of importance to people in the group. We decided therefore to use the collective term 'staff' for all people who worked with them and to draw up two lists, one of things they thought staff should do and the other of things they thought staff shouldn't do.

One of the tutors from the learning difficulties degree met with the group for three consecutive weeks for an hour. Group members responded enthusiastically to the task. They were pleased and proud to have been asked to help. They had a great deal to say about how they thought staff should behave towards them. Notes were made by the tutor as they were speaking and the two lists were drawn up. These were revised on a week-by-week basis until all members of the group were happy with them. The lists, which are reproduced in Table 1.1, have been used each year since then to prepare the Level Two degree students for placement.

Table 1.1 The lists of 'shoulds' and 'shouldn'ts'

Staff should
- Be patient
- Be understanding
- Understand about embarrassing things like monthly periods
- Spend time getting to know us and any difficulties we might have
- Help us sort our problems out
- Listen to us and let us finish what we are saying
- Have time for us
- Let us do things in our own time
- Let us go to bed early if we want to
- Believe us if we say we are ill
- Help us keep in touch with our friends
- Let us leave early if we want to
- Ask us if we are happy about having a support worker of the opposite sex

Staff should not
- Have one rule for them and another rule for us
- Say we are overweight if we're not allowed to say they're overweight
- Tell us our clothes are creased if we're not allowed to tell them their clothes are creased
- Say things like 'only babies go to bed early'
- Block their ears
- Push or pull us
- Bully us
- Tell us off like a child
- Call us 'spastic' or 'brain damaged'
- Talk about us as if we are not there

The degree students are usually shocked by the intensity of the lists, particularly the issue of time and people's concern about having to accept personal care from a support worker of the opposite sex. Even though the lists were prepared some time ago, each year they are revisited the degree students have little difficulty in citing current examples firmly located on the 'staff should not' list.

References

Barron, D. (1996) *A Price to be Born*, Harrogate, Mencap Northern Division.

Part II

The context of learning disability services

Chapter 2

The historical context

David Race

Introduction

As a young PhD student writing nearly twenty-five years ago on the historical development of service provision, I started my account with the following somewhat naive statement:

> Unlike other physiological or biochemical disorders, such as damaged limbs, which have been observed and classified to something approaching an agreed level, mental disorder, and specifically mental handicap, has been subject to wide disagreements among those connected with it. These disagreements, in fact, go beyond classification, and on to causation, prognosis, and the most acceptable method of treatment. The mere use of the term 'mental handicap' immediately places the author into a certain sector of this spectrum of opinion, whereas the use of alternatives such as mental subnormality, mental retardation, mental deficiency etc., would have located him elsewhere.
>
> (Race 1977 : 3)

Plus ça change . . . with the addition of a few more terms in the last part, such as intellectual impairment, learning disability, or learning difficulties, and an acknowledgement that the 'agreement' in the first part of the statement has been seriously challenged by the disability movement, the overall argument would, I contend, still hold true. What *has* changed in those twenty-five years, as this and other chapters will elaborate, is the identity of those parties 'connected with' the issue, the nature of the 'disagreements', and the power to influence change of the various protagonists. In addition, from a relatively simple and finite number of parties to the debate (with some, indeed, being reluctant participants) there now exists a veritable tower of Babel of views on service issues, and subsets of service issues, so that the student seeking enlightenment as to why services are as they are is faced with a bewildering mass of information. Some of this could be said to be 'empirical' (though see the discussion in Chapter 7), some emphatically not, being statements of values concerning things such as 'rights', and much, as Sydney Smith remarked on the two women shouting at each other from their respective front doors, finding no common ground, as they were 'arguing from different premises'.

Such is the cacophony of these disagreements that one might expect services to be in a constant state of change, with swings between the different 'fashions' bringing this year's set of emperor's new clothes to the fore, and last year's cast-offs going to the charity shop. A glance at the many sets of procedures and (some-times) books that reside on the shelves of the offices of a number of services would reinforce this view. Here will be the Individual Programme Plan manual, there the PASS or PASSING manual (usually in the offices of service managers of a certain age); here again the video on PATH or MAPS, and there the Personal Lifestyle Planning Documentation. Then those with a more medical bent may have works on dealing with challenging behaviour, or 'active support'. What is less likely to be as variable, even at the beginning of the millennium, is the physical location of the service, the numbers of people served, the qualifications of those providing the services, and the range of abilities and identities of those using the services. The Department of Health survey, *Facing the Facts* (1999) (covered in more detail in Chapter 7), confirmed what had been an impression for some time, that in the nearly thirty years since the document *Better Services for the Mentally Handicapped* (DHSS 1971) much debate had taken place, many changes had been made in moving people from large institutions, many books had been written documenting those changes, and yet

> it was striking that congregate forms of care still predominated, with two thirds of people accommodated in some form of congregate living arrangement, and two thirds still using block day services such as Adult Training Centres or Social Education Centres.
>
> (DoH 1999: 3)

So is there something more deep-rooted in the way in which services for people with learning difficulties have been conceived? Why have we ended up with the services we have? I would contend that there are a number of key factors to be gleaned from the history of services that are highly relevant to attempts at answering those questions. The first of these is the inextricable link between the classification of people and the sorts of responses, including services, to that classification.

Early classifications and responses

In a controversial but fascinating presentation (Wolfensberger 2000, as yet unpub-lished), Wolf Wolfensberger traces the vast number of words in the Indo-European group of languages that refer to what was commonly called 'natural stupidity'. His thesis is that, as shown by the development of language and through evidence from representations in iconography and art, ordinary people had a clear understanding of who fell into the category of 'natural fools', i.e. those whose condition was from birth or immediately surrounding birth. This is supported by the distinction, ironically increasingly blurred in modern discourse, especially the written press, between those people who would be now described as having mental health problems and those described as having learning difficulties. Matthews (1954) quotes a statute of 1325 (De praerogativa regis) which dealt differently with the lands of an 'idiot' and a 'lunatic'. 'Idiots' (i.e. 'natural fools') were to have their lands protected, their necessities provided for, and their lands passed to the proper heirs on their death. 'Lunatics' (i.e. persons of unsound mind) had their lands protected so that they might be restored to them on their recovery. The difference between the two was thus seen to be the permanence of the condition and the possibility of 'reason' returning. John Locke, the philosopher, summed it up as follows. Quoted in Hilliard and Kirman (1965) he concluded that:

> In short herein seems to be the difference between Idiots and Madmen, that Madmen put wrong ideas together, and so make wrong propositions, but argue and reason right from them, but Idiots make very few or no propositions and reason scarce at all.
>
> (Locke 1689)

The importance Locke attaches to 'reason' was, of course, part of the growing movement, at least in the relatively small intellectual, religious and aristocratic circles of Europe, towards seeing the human, and the human intellect, as being the centre of all earthly activity and purpose, replacing the 'superstitious' religion where God held that place. That movement, usually called the 'Enlightenment' had many ramifications, (see e.g. Tawney 1938) but for people with learning difficulties these would not be fully realised until they were combined with another key event in European history.

The Industrial Revolution, like the Enlightenment, had many effects that are still with us today, but for the group of people we are concerned with its importance is, I would contend, major. Prior to the Industrial Revolution, as we have seen, there was a clear view of who were 'natural fools' and also a fairly common view of what was appropriate behaviour towards them. Most of this was relatively benign tolerance, and even in some cases a valuing of what were seen as unique gifts of 'fools'. An example is the case of 'court fools', who would be given fairly valued roles in court circles, as a reminder to the monarch of his human frailty when he started getting too full of his own importance. For the great majority, however, in the rural economy of the pre-Industrial Revolution period, the possession of a limited intellectual ability had no particular significance. Even people who would today be definitely identified as people with learning difficulties, such as those with Down's syndrome, could have a part to play as the 'village idiot' and could certainly be actively helpful in the predominantly manual work involved in rural life. Those who would today fall at the 'less severe' end of classification would not be regarded as 'natural fools' and in fact would probably not be distinguishable, or distinguished in the public mind, from the rest of the population, since the vast majority of that population could not read or write, and were not usually called upon to make many decisions involving detailed intellectual reasoning, or to carry out highly skilled work.

With the Enlightenment, however, came the growth in calls for education, and with the Industrial Revolution came the process of urbanisation and a need for skills, albeit at a basic level, to survive in the mill or factory. This began to mark out a further group of people as of low ability and employability. When combined with an increasingly utilitarian approach to the centuries old laws for relief of the poor in parishes throughout the country, exemplified in the Poor Law Amendment Act of 1834 and the setting up of 'workhouses', a gradual change was set in train. Not so much in public services, which were few in number anyway, but in attitudes and beliefs about what it was to be human, and what constituted a person's place on the scale of humanness. Again, it is easy with hindsight to condemn those responsible for the development of asylums and workhouses, and the division of people into the 'deserving' and 'undeserving' poor, but it should be borne in mind how small, even a mere 150 years ago, were the numbers of people in positions of power over communities, how few people moved more than a short distance from their native village or town, and how limited was most people's education, at least in the terms that we would now understand it. Leaders of opinion therefore also tended to be leaders of communities in the power sense of that word, and as such their views on the nature of humanity, and the poor and dependent, led to the very prescribed nature of life in the workhouse, with conditions being set as a deterrent to people to enter, rather than any effort at making their lives comfortable (Owen 1965).

Ironically this contrasts, to some extent at least, with conditions in the asylums. One of the more positive things to come from the Enlightenment, at least as compared with later attitudes, was a belief in the possibility of development through education. Again, the relatively small number of people in academic and intellectual circles at the turn of the nineteenth century should be borne in mind, and therefore the relative ease with which 'discoveries' could be disseminated, together with the much greater range of subjects covered by any one man (and it was at that point almost totally men). Thus when the French educationalist Itard published an account in 1801 of his meeting and teaching the 'Wild boy of Aveyron' it quickly reached this circle of 'renaissance men.' Itard's account told of meeting a youth running wild in the woods on all fours like his animal companions and with no speech other than animal-like noises. By taking the boy to his home, gaining his trust and attention, and spending a lot of time in individual contact with him, Itard was able to teach him rudimentary skills and some speech. Itard's pupil Seguin took his theories further and proposed that 'idiots' and 'imbeciles' had the use of their intellectual faculties but lacked the power to apply them because of a lack of resistance to competing stimuli. This also accords with Wolfensberger's (2000) observation of what was commonly held about 'natural fools' – that they lacked judgement, were easily led, but could learn simple things through imitation. Itard's and then Seguin's basic technique was thus to attract and then keep their pupil's attention, restrict the competing stimuli, and therefore instil the skills through constant reinforcement. Pioneering institutions, such as those set up by Guggenbuhl in Switzerland and Reed in England were thus designed not to keep people away from the world, as they most definitely were later, but to keep the world away from them, so that they would not be distracted from their 'training and education'.

We therefore have a fairly optimistic view, at least in educational circles, as the nineteenth century progressed, and this was, of course, matched by pressure for more universal education in society as a whole, reflected in the various Royal Commissions which eventually led to the large number of schools that were in place by the end of that century, Owen (1965). For people with learning difficulties, the Idiots Act of 1886 set up a duty on Local Authorities to provide 'care, education and training' in special asylums. In some cases this continued the educational ethos of the earlier institutions. In others, a mixture of confused terminology in an earlier act, the Lunatic Asylums Act of 1853, and the ever-increasing parsimony of public services, meant that both 'idiots' and 'lunatics' were served in the same asylum or they were both, along with the poor, the elderly and the physically impaired, placed all together in the workhouse. Again, we need to remember that people in such places were still in a considerable minority, with most simply living in the villages and towns where they were born, with as great variation in tolerance as those places contained variation in people. In addition, as we have also noted, those called 'idiots' were a much more clearly identified group. As the school system increased, and the factories to fuel the empire demanded more workers with manual skills and dexterity, more people began to be identified as 'lacking'. When put alongside that other great product of the Enlightenment, the rise of Darwinism and eugenics, the stage was set for a major change in attitudes and provision to the expanding range of people who were beginning to be grouped under the heading of 'mentally deficient'.

The eugenic alarm and the growth of 'colonies'

As well as being marked out by the developing school system as of limited academic ability, the group of people at the bottom of the fully developed and powerful class system of the late Victorian era were also subject to increasingly moral approbation from society. Ironically, in that the former was later to effectively replace Judeo-Christianity as a de facto religion, the combination of the rise of science and the moralising tone of social policymakers at the turn of the twentieth century brought together two previously distinct groups under one heading, where they were to remain, with little real change, to the present day. Prior to the last decade of the nineteenth century, the group who became known as the 'feeble-minded' had scarcely been thought of as a distinct category of people. Those who now fell into that category had previously been described in various ways as 'lazy', 'feckless', 'idle', 'wicked', 'sturdy beggars', and so on (Thane 1982). Now, the growing impact of Darwinism on the study of human beings, led by, among others, Francis Galton and Julian Huxley, increasingly saw the behaviour of such people as evidence of an inherent defect of mind, or 'feeblemindedness', that could be put alongside the centuries old common understanding of the identity of 'natural fools'.

Indeed, some of the benevolent attitudes in the asylums for the latter group could be found in the setting up of charitable institutions for the 'care and education of the feebleminded' (Tredgold 1922).

The classification became sufficiently established in the (still very small) academic and policymaking circles as to be included as a separate category in the census of 1901, resulting in the reporting of some 13,000 cases. Given the far more arbitrary nature of this classification, which depended very largely on behaviour that went against the prevailing norms of society, it is scarcely surprising that the numbers of such people were seen to be increasing. This, in turn, was supported by many learned 'scientific' papers (e.g. Pearson and Jaederholm 1914) purporting to show the inevitable rise in the 'feebleminded' population and the 'danger' this posed to society. A Royal Commission, set up in 1904 to make recommendations as to the 'care of the feebleminded', soon requested that its remit be extended to cover all forms of mental disorder, including 'idiots' and 'lunatics'.

One of the Commission's key members was A.F. Tredgold, described in his books as a 'Lecturer in Mental Deficiency' at London University, but also 'Physician to the Outpatient Department at Bethlem Royal Hospital'. He was one of an increasingly powerful group who came together under the general heading of those concerned with 'eugenics'. The word was coming into common usage and was the product of two factors which, in the view of Tizard (1958: 3), who was himself to become highly influential on service development in the 1960s and 1970s, 'set the service back by fifty years'. These were the extension, already alluded to, of Darwinist ideas into the developing science of 'genetics' and the development, by Binet in Paris, of a standardised instrument to measure something called 'intelligence'. The idea of an inherited intellectual ability, which is unaltered by training or education, and in fact determines one's response to education or training, was not new at the beginning of the twentieth century, but was somewhat in a minority. The combination, however, of genetic 'findings' on the inheritability of many characteristics, beyond physiological ones such as eye colour, and the arrival of a supposedly 'scientific measure' of intelligence persuaded many in academic circles of the invariance of this 'inherent ability'. Current popular debates about 'designer babies' and the 'gene for' this or that desirable or undesirable condition have, of course, their roots in this discussion, as have current policies to 'screen out' disabled people their roots in developments which followed the Royal Commission's report in 1908.

The first of these developments was the recommendation to group together the various disparate categories mentioned above into one classification, to be called 'mental defect' or 'mental deficiency'. This, among other things, exacerbated the confusion, which continues to this day, between mental health and learning disability, and gave further credence to the 'inheritability' thesis by associating those whose condition had always been known to exist from birth or early age (the 'natural fools') with those where this had not really been demonstrated ('the feebleminded'). The classificatory grouping was then used, in intense debates within the still small group of academics and policymakers, to press for changes to the law to deal with the 'problem' of mental deficiency. Tredgold published the first edition of his *Textbook on Mental Deficiency* in the same year as the Royal Commission reported. This textbook was to run to thirteen editions, five after Tredgold's death, and was used in medical training up until the mid-1980s. Tredgold then went on, in 1909, to publish a famous paper in the *Eugenics Review* where he outlined the views that were to become the backbone of the legislation which followed. His view, widely supported, was that:

> as soon as a nation reaches that stage of civilisation in which medical knowledge and humanitarian sentiment operate to prolong the existence of the unfit, then it becomes imperative upon that nation to devise such social laws as will ensure that those unfit do not propagate their kind.
>
> (Tredgold 1909: 8)

Before we become too harsh in our hindsight judgement of these views, let us consider the operation of the Abortion (Amendment) Act of 1992, still the law as this is written. As Morris (1991) points out, the fact that only children with disabilities are allowed by this law to be aborted up to term reproduces a policy of society not to 'prolong the existence of the unfit'. Termination of life was, in fact a policy which Tredgold was later to advocate, as we shall discuss below, but at the time of his 1909 article he was proposing a less final, but nevertheless devastating, way of removing people from society.

> 1. In the first place the chief evil we have to prevent is undoubtedly that of propagation. 2. Next, society must be protected against such of these persons as either have definite criminal tendencies, or are of so facile a disposition that they readily commit crimes at the instigation of others. 3. Lastly, even where these poor creatures are relatively harmless, we have to protect society from the burden due to their non-productiveness.
>
> (Tredgold 1909: 3)

Thus all the bogeys that bedevil people to this day come at once. People are a menace, a burden, and what is more they are propagating at a greater rate. Again, students should look at current utterances about certain groups of people, particularly in the tabloid press, and discern their origins. Tredgold goes on to propose his solution, which was taken up, after some debate in Parliament, as the main policy thrust of the Mental Deficiency Act of 1913.

> I have come to the conclusion that, in the case of the majority of the feebleminded, there is one measure, and one measure only, which will fulfil all these desiderata and which is at the same time practically possible, namely the establishment of suitable industrial and farm colonies . . . Society would thus be saved a portion, at least, of the cost of their maintenance, and, more

important, it would be secure from their depredation and danger of their propagation.

(Tregold 1909.: 7)

The Act itself, as noted, set up the processes by which people could be detained and, more importantly to this chapter, the definition of who was a 'mental defective'. This can be summarised as follows, and it is important to note that the 1913 Act, and therefore the definition of who was a 'mental defective', was to remain in force for nearly half a century. The institutions in which people so classified were segregated were to last much longer.

The Act classified 'defectives' under four headings.

1   Idiots – these were people who were 'so deeply defective in mind from birth or from early age as to be unable to guard themselves against common physical dangers'.
2   Imbeciles – these were persons who, whilst not as defective as idiots, were still incapable of 'managing their own affairs'.
3   Feebleminded persons – these were persons who were not as defective as imbeciles but required 'care, supervision and control for their own protection or for the protection of others'.
4   Moral defectives – these were persons who 'from an early age display some permanent mental defect coupled with strong vicious or criminal propensities on which punishment has had little or no effect'.

The language of these definitions, it hardly needs pointing out, reveals how much more of a social issue is the subject of learning disability than a medical one. All definitions are written in terms which describe the *effect* of the so-called defect rather than any empirically measurable definition of what the defect actually *is*, and all contain descriptive statements which are totally bound up with the transitory norms and understandings of a particular society. We have already seen how the Industrial Revolution, with its need for manual skills and dexterity, and the Enlightenment view of the dominance of reason and the human mind had led to a whole extra category of people being classed as 'failing' those criteria. A moment's study should reveal to the reader contemporary conditions and groups of people who would likewise 'fail' to 'manage their own affairs' or who could be described as requiring 'care, supervision and control', or as having 'vicious or criminal propensities'. They would not, however, only include those falling under the classi-fication of 'learning disability' and some who currently fall under that classification would not fit any of the categories of the 1913 Act. The point is that society's concern for maintaining itself (or at least those who have positions of power in that society) creates those it wishes to segregate.

The processes of the 1913 Act reinforce the point. Section Two gives the conditions under which a person 'who was a defective' might be dealt with by being sent to an institution for defectives (increasingly, and interestingly in view of the other contemporary usage of the word, being called 'colonies'):

a) At the instance of his parent or guardian.

b) If in addition to being a defective he was a person
   i) who was found neglected, abandoned, or without visible means of support, or cruelly treated or . . . in need of care or training which could not be provided in his home; or
   ii) who was found guilty of any criminal offence, or who was ordered to be sent to an approved school; or
   iii) who was undergoing imprisonment, or was in an approved school; or
   iv) who was an habitual drunkard; or
   v) who had been found incapable of receiving education at school, or that by reason of disability of mind might require supervision after leaving school.

If a parent or guardian was attempting to place their child in an institution they required two medical certificates from qualified medical practitioners, one of whom was approved for the purpose by the local health authority or the Minister of Health. The other reasons for a 'defective' being sent to an institution, i.e. those under b) above, could be cited by any number of people, such as relatives, friends, neighbours, or a Local Authority officer, in a petition to a 'judicial authority' again accompanied by two medical certificates. Institutions were under a Board of Control and ultimately responsible to the Local Authority, and it was this Board that made decisions on the admission and continuing detention of 'defectives'. Notice the need for 'medical certificates', which not only places power of diagnosis in the hands of doctors, a power retained to this day in many respects, but also gives them the power over where a person might go, and the power to keep them there. Even today, doctors' certificates are required by many countries, even of perfectly healthy people with learning difficulties, in order for them to travel abroad. So though the 'colonies' were not staffed, in the main, by doctors and nurses, the 'medical model' referred to by modern disability activists, e.g. Oliver (1990), was firmly in place in terms of power over who got to be called a 'defective'.

Over the ensuing twenty to thirty years the effects of being so classified were also fairly similar. In England and Wales numbers of 'defectives' under the 'care and control' of the Mental Deficiency Act rose from 12,000 in 1920, through 37,000 in 1926, to 90,000 by 1939, with growth levelling off to give a figure of 100,000 by 1950 (Tredgold 1952). As O'Connor (1965) notes, 'the tendency to build large institutions for about 2,000 patients in isolated country areas was a definite policy'. He might have added that parsimony by Local Authorities also brought the conversion of large numbers of workhouses, lunatic asylums and former TB sanatoria into the category of 'suitable institutions'.

The Wood Report, the results of another commission to examine the amount and type of education required for 'mental defectives', sums up the official version of conditions with frightening clarity:

the modern institution is generally a large one, preferably built on a colony plan, takes defectives of all grades of defect and of all ages. All, of course are properly classified according to their mental capacity and age. The Local Mental Deficiency Authority have to provide for all grades of defect, all types of case and all ages, and an institution that cannot, or will not, take this case for one reason and that case for another is of no use to the Authority. An institution which takes all types and ages is economical because the high-grade patients do the work and make everything necessary, not only for themselves, but also for the lower grade. In an institution taking only lower grades, the whole of the work has to be done by paid staff; in one taking only high grades the output of the work is greater than that required for the institution itself and there is difficulty in disposing of it. In the all-grade institution, on the other hand, the high-grade patients are the skilled workmen of the colony, those who do all the higher processes of manufacture, those on whom there is a considerable measure of responsibility; the medium grade patients are the labourers, who do the more simple routine work in the training shops and about the institution; the best of the lower-grade patients fetch and carry or do the very simple work.

(Wood Report 1929: 33)

As before, too harsh a modern view of the sentiments expressed above should be tempered with both a clear understanding of the values and beliefs of societies in the period in question, and also an analysis of contemporary utterances and even some policies regarding the need for 'the disabled' to be provided with 'work for those who can and help for those who cannot'.

The eugenic views that had led to the Mental Deficiency Act and the setting up of 'colonies' were not confined to academic thought in the UK. Throughout the USA and Europe, as economies recovered from the first war and then suffered the effects of the Great Depression of the 1920s and 1930s (Thane 1982), utilitarian views on 'productiveness' of individuals and their 'costs to society' were brought into sharp focus. In Germany the coming to power of Hitler and his particular spin on racial purity added to an already strong view in European academic circles regarding what to do with people whose lives, as described in the title of one influential academic paper, were 'devoid of value' (Binding and Hoche 1920).

What then took place in Germany, with the so-called *euthanasie* programme providing the blueprint for what was to come later in the 'final solution' of the Holocaust, has only been fully explored by academics much later (Lifton 1986; Annas 1992). In this programme, those classified as 'incurably mentally ill' were sent to so-called 'hospitals' which were, in fact, places where they were killed, initially in gas chambers and latterly by lethal injection. Though hidden from the general public, the programme was well publicised within the Nazi party and in the realms of academia. It also appears to have been known about in other parts of Europe, including the UK, and really represented a carrying out of policies equally stongly advocated in those countries. As late as the eighth (1952) edition of his textbook, Tredgold's views are clear, and he was far from unique. Speaking of the '80,000 or more idiots or imbeciles in this country' he writes:

> These are not only incapable of being employed to any economic advantage, but their care and support, whether in their own homes or in institutions, absorb a large amount of time, energy and money of the normal population which could be utilised to better purpose. Moreover, many of these defectives are utterly helpless, repulsive in appearance, and revolting in manners. Their existence is a perpetual source of sorrow and unhappiness to their parents, and those who live at home have a most disturbing influence upon other children and family life. With the present shortage of institutional accommodation there are thousands of mothers who are literally worn out in caring for these persons at home. In my opinion it would be an economical and humane procedure were their existence to be painlessly terminated.
>
> (Tredgold 1952: 92)

That Tredgold was still able to present these views post-war, even as the full horror of the Holocaust was being revealed, shows the lack of connection made between it and the *euthanasie* programme, the virtual silence on the latter at Nuremberg, and the general agreement on such views within the academic community.

Same places, different names – absorption into the National Health Service

There appears to have been some debate within the government and civil service as to the place of the colonies in the newly created 'Welfare State' that the incoming Labour government set in train after 1945 (Sullivan 1992). The difficulty that the minister in charge, Anaurin Bevan, had in persuading the medical profession to accept the idea of a National Health Service seems to have reduced the fate of the colonies to an afterthought (Thane 1982). Though usually possessed of a 'medical superintendent', such as the dynasty of Langdon Down at Normansfield in Surrey, the colonies had been a Local Authority responsibility, and had largely been staffed by untrained and unqualified members of the community around them. Indeed, because of their size and remoteness, the colonies were sometimes the major employer in certain localities, with employment being passed down the generations as in mining communities. Now, with the decision finally being to incorporate them into the new NHS, 'colonies' became 'hospitals' overnight and trainee nurses, administrators and doctors would receive in their studies the accumulated wisdom and values of forty years of segregation, including, as virtually the only major textbook of its day, a further five editions of Tredgold's *Mental Deficiency*. The effect of this move, with its concomitant inclusion of all grades of nursing, medical and ancillary staff into the common pay scales, hierarchies, training and budgetary systems of the NHS, cannot be overemphasised. To the time of writing, the power of what others have termed a 'medical model' of service has been maintained in

the world of learning disability services. Despite all the hospital closures, government reports, incentives and even legislation to try and get either joint working
with others, or others as 'lead authorities', power over the learning disability agenda
(even the 'official' adoption of that classification) has remained in the hands of the
Department of Health.

The current ramifications of that situation are discussed in other chapters, but as
far as the post-war period was concerned, the pessimism and negativity so
powerfully expressed by Tredgold remained the dominant ethos. Within the new
NHS, too, the field of learning disability was not one to which doctors and nurses
flocked. Though on the same salary scales as other consultants, those training in
psychiatry, itself a relatively unpopular option, would tend to go far more readily
for the mental illness field, particularly as the new 'pharmacological straightjacket'
of mind drugs was fertile ground for their clinical skills. This tended to result,
through a combination of market forces in personnel and conscious or unconscious
racism within the medical selection processes, in a disproportionate representation
of doctors and nurses from the euphemistically described 'New Commonwealth'
within learning disability hospitals in certain parts of the country (Martin 1984).

In education, too, the 1944 Education Act, set up with some considerable
influence from Cyril Burt, a leading advocate of the 'innate intelligence' school,
had continued to define a class of children as 'incapable' of receiving education at
school. These 'ineducable' children, defined as such by the IQ tests that were also
the basis of the selection of children at 'eleven plus', for the prestige of the
'grammar schools' or the perceived failure of a 'secondary modern school', had
no schools at all to attend. Controversy over the 'eleven plus', however, over-
shadowed the small voice of the embryonic National Society for Mentally
Handicapped Children in seeking to get education for their offspring (see Chapter
4 for the continuing ramifications of that campaign). In addition, of course, there
were still considerable numbers of children residing permanently in the hospitals,
for whom no formal education was thought necessary.

For parents of a child with learning difficulties then, the 1950s and 1960s
presented very similar options to pre-war. They could take what was usually the
advice on the birth of a child with an obvious condition, such as Down's syndrome,
to 'leave them here, and let the NHS look after them' or they could raise the child,
without a school to send them to, and with only the hospital as an alternative if
this became impossible. Tredgold's remarks about 'worn out mothers' certainly
had some validity.

At an academic level, most of the developments of the 1950s and 1960s that
in any way challenged the dominant medical pessimism came from the growing
field of psychology. The work of Tizard, O'Connor and the Clarkes formed
the vanguard of a number of studies concerning the potential of 'mental defectives'
and the higher than expected IQ levels to be found amongst inmates of the hospitals.
O'Connor and Tizard (1954) and Clarke and Clarke (1953, 1954) are three
examples, and for a fuller list see Race (1977). With the backing of their own studies,
therefore, researchers were not only demonstrating the potential of people but were

criticising, either implicitly or explicitly, the institutional regimes in operation. Later studies began to look specifically at the link between living environments and IQ, e.g. Clarke *et.al.* (1958), Kirk (1958), and therefore the view, expressed by Gunzburg (1957), that the hospital should ideally exist as some sort of rehabilitation centre, preparing people for community living, began to establish itself, especially among what could be called the 'psychologists group'.

Despite these views, however, their transmission into any sort of change in the minds of those actually providing hospital services in the 1950s and 1960s was not particularly marked. In the early part of that period, a Royal Commission was set up to review the law 'relating to Mental Illness and Mental Deficiency', not really as an attempt at positive change in the underlying assumption of the need for institutions, but as a response to a few well-publicised cases of wrongful detention, mainly in psychiatric hospitals. The subsequent legislation, therefore, though it changed the terminology from the 1914 Act, did little to alter conditions in the hospitals.

The 1959 Mental Health Act did at least remove the 'moral defective' category from its new terminology, in fact insisting, in Section 4, that 'Nothing in this section shall be construed as implying that a person may be dealt with . . . by reason only of promiscuity or other immoral conduct'. The preceding part of Section 4, however, did little to remove the confusion, referred to earlier, between learning disability and mental health, and in fact created a further categorisation that was to last another twenty years at least. It is reproduced in full below:

1) In this Act 'mental disorder' means mental illness, arrested or incomplete development of mind, psychopathic disorder, and any other disorder or disability of mind; and 'mentally disordered' shall be construed accordingly.

2) In this Act 'severe subnormality' means a state of arrested or incomplete development of mind which includes subnormality of intelligence and is of such a nature or degree that the patient is incapable of living an independent life or of guarding himself against serious exploitation, or will be incapable when of an age to do so.

3) In this Act 'subnormality' means a state of arrested or incomplete development of mind (not amounting to severe subnormality) which includes subnormality of intelligence and is of a nature or degree which requires or is susceptible to medical treatment or other special care or training of the patient.

4) In this Act 'psychopathic disorder' means a persistent disorder or disability of mind (whether or not including subnormality of intelligence) which results in abnormally aggressive or seriously irresponsible conduct on the part of the patient, and requires, or is susceptible to, medical treatment.

(Mental Health Act 1959)

As with its predecessor of forty-six years, the definitions are again essentially subjective and essentially related to contemporary norms of behaviour. What is added, however, is the clear footprint of the medical model, in the use of words like 'patient' and the predominant position of 'medical treatment' as the 'need' of this category of person. There is also no definition of what constitutes 'subnormality of intelligence' either in terms of IQ levels or even in terms of any particular intelligence 'measure'. Classification in practice, therefore, remained in the hands of those doing the defining, no longer predominantly GPs, but now the growing number of consultant psychiatrists and clinical psychologists that inclusion in the NHS had brought to the former 'colonies'.

Debates and scandals – the beginnings of community care

In academic circles, both in the UK and in the increasingly influential USA, the studies of the 'psychologists group' continued to cast doubt on the inadequacy of an IQ classification. Castell and Mittler (1965), for example, contrasted the views of twenty hospitals on what constituted 'subnormality' and 'severe subnormality' in terms of IQ with their own IQ measurements of people so classified, and found considerable disparities. Such research tied in with a number of 'follow-up studies', especially those carried out in the USA by Baller, Charles and Miller (1967), that showed earlier classifications to have considerably underestimated the abilities of people called 'defectives', and led to a search, at least in those academic circles, for some sort of 'scientific' measure of 'adaptive behaviour' or 'social competence'. In some quarters, especially the USA, this was only to set one measure alongside another, given the existing heavy professional commitment to the IQ test, and led to the development and adoption of various scales, most notably those of Nihara and his colleagues (Nihara *et al.* 1969). In others, the focus on the unrecognised ability of people to acquire skills, and the success of 'experiments' where, given adequate training and a stimulating environment, such skills could be developed (Claridge 1961; Clarke and Blakemore 1961; Gunzburg 1961) gave something of a contrast to the still strongly segregationist views of the medical establishment. This latter group, particularly the Mental Deficiency section of the Royal College of Psychiatrists, viewed with alarm the planned number of 'hostels' in the ten-year plan for England and Wales (Ministry of Health 1962), though the definition of such places only consisted of them being described as 'small units'and no really settled 'model' existed for their design. The ten-year plan came at the time when a young Enoch Powell was Minister of Health, as part of a Conservative government going into its eleventh year of office, and in what Jones *et al.* (1979) describe as a 'somewhat intemperate speech' in 1961 he announced 'the run down of the mental hospital'. Though Jones calls this a 'real shift of emphasis', it should be noted in relation to our subject that the speech concerned all the long-stay groups in hospital, not just people with learning difficulties. Equally, the publication of the so-called Blue Book *Health and Welfare: the Development of Community Care* (Ministry of Health 1963), though it may have been one of the earliest official uses of the term, gave only very general advice to

Local Authorities, and had no earmarked funding for the so-called 'development'. Where Jones may well be right, however, in the significance of this speech is in the analysis of the political motivation behind it, not least the desire to reduce public spending. It is interesting to compare the motivations behind the NHS and Community Care Act, nearly thirty years later, also brought in by a Conservative government in its eleventh year in power, and to observe the prescience of Professor Richard Titmuss, in opposing Powell's speech on the grounds that the 'primary motive was economic'. This is covered in greater detail in Chapter 6 but in terms of developments in learning disability services other events were to push the debate forwards. The combined effects of further demonstrations of the effects of environments, both negative and positive, from the 'psychologists group' together with a number of well-publicised scandals and a particularly active minister in Richard Crossman brought to the fore the more positive view of the development of services expressed in the 1971 White Paper, *Better Services for the Mentally Handicapped* (and, incidentally, the growing use of the term 'mental handicap' itself).

As early as 1964, Tizard had made out the case for 'an approach to the problem of organising residential care for the mentally subnormal which is based on small residential units, closely associated with the day care services of a particular area'. This, in his view, could cover all 'grades of defect' and replace the hospital-oriented approach, with nursing care only being provided for chair and bed-fast patients. Others, especialy Gunzburg, continued the call for more intensive training of people with learning difficulties, and developments in Adult Training Centres of 'work based training' had their successes (Moorman 1967, Price 1967, Williams 1967). These debates, however, though they were important, did not appear to be shifting the power of the hospitals significantly.

In 1967, the *News of the World* (then, as now, investigating 'scandal' though with slightly more words than currently employed) carried a story about abuse at Ely hospital in Cardiff. This had come from a 'whistle-blowing' nurse and was to lead to a public inquiry, headed by a young Conservative MP and barrister Geoffrey Howe. The minister in the then Labour government, Richard Crossman, reveals in his diaries (Crossman 1977) that senior civil servants at the Department of Health and Social Security were not only aware of conditions at Ely, but also knew that conditions were little different in hospitals elsewhere. Crossman also gives a fascinating account of attempts to keep the Howe Report (1969) out of the public domain and his own efforts to improve the conditions of hospitals.

At the same time, two major studies, one by a sociologist and one by psychologists, added yet further academic weight to the call for changes in care. Pauline Morris's 1969 sociological study of conditions in thirty-five subnormality hospitals was highly critical of conditions therein, and gave the broadest picture then produced of those conditions. It not only included criticisms of the direct work with patients, finding few medical needs, virtually no assessment of need, and few objectives for patients other than containment, but also had strong words to say on the physical conditions, the small and untrained workforce, and on the poor, even hostile, communication between staff of various levels and between the hospitals and the outside world.

The second study, by psychologists from the Institute of Education in London led by Tizard, contained the same indictment of the hospital system. Using a typology developed from Goffman's *Asylums* (1961), fast becoming the bible of the anti-institution movement in both the USA and UK, Tizard and his team studied services for children with learning difficulties in various residential settings (King and Raynes, 1968; Raynes and King, 1968; King *et al.* 1971). They identified four 'interrelated characteristics' of the hospital pattern of care: rigidity of routine; 'block' treatment; depersonalisation; and 'social distance' between staff and children. The authors found that this pattern of care contrasted sharply with the approach of the Local Authority hostels for children. Voluntary homes had a greater variation, falling along a spectrum between the hospitals and the hostels.

Radicalism or paternalism? – the 1971 White Paper

These pieces of research, along with Crossman's response to the hospital scandals, clearly had some effect. In the short term, there were improvements in the physical appearance of some hospitals, with so-called 'Crossman units' appearing in hospital grounds and the old wards being smartened up. Crossman also set up a Hospital Advisory Service, reporting direct to the minister out of the clutches of the civil servants. These were, however, only put into place in the final years of a Labour government, and it was left to Crossman's Conservative successor, Keith Joseph, to publish in 1971 the White Paper which represented the policy development of the activities of the 1960s. Entitled *Better Services for the Mentally Handicapped* the document has a number of elements that indicate thinking well ahead of contemporary practice, and more in line with the relatively radical academics, led by Tizard in terms of influence, that we have just reviewed.

The use of the term 'mental handicap' is justified in the White Paper 'in preference to any of the alternative terms because this helps to emphasise that our attitude should be the same as to other types of handicap' (DHSS 1971: 1). This new classification owed something to the pressure brought to bear by the National Society for Mentally Handicapped Children to spread the term 'mental handicap' into common usage, though 'subnormality' remained the legal term. This was one of a number of achievements claimed by the National Society at the time. By achieving the recognition of a right to education of all children in the Education (Handicapped Children) Act of 1970, the National Society had realised one of its major campaigning goals, and, in its sponsorship of the 'Slough Experiment' (Baranjay 1971) it had also demonstrated the 'radical' alternative to hospital provision in the form of the hostel. Though radical for its day, however, the National Society's roots as a parents' movement made a challenge to the overall attitude of paternalism inherent in the medical model unlikely, as the disability movement have pointed out (Barnes 1997). It was therefore caught up in what appeared to many parents to be a whirlwind of change, and debates in local branches of the National Society showed serious divisions over the White Paper (National Society for Mentally Handicapped Children (NSMHC) 1974).

Divisions appeared elsewhere, too. For those on the radical end of the spectrum (Campaign for the Mentally Handicapped (CMH), 1971; 1972) the proposals were considered half-hearted and lacking any real sense of effective change. Whilst advocating a dramatic fall in the number of hospital places for adults from roughly 90 per cent of residential provision to 40 per cent the White Paper did not really explain why the remaining 40 per cent were needed, nor why the alternative should be the hostel. The psychiatrists group, on the other hand, criticised the fact that their responsibilities were being diminished in response to 'unqualified' pressure (Royal Medico-Psychological Association 1971).

Alongside these debates, however, broader policy initiatives were having their effect. The report of the Seebohm Committee (Home Office *et al.* 1968) and the subsequent legislation setting up 'generic' Social Services Departments included 'social care' of people with learning difficulties in their remit. The new departments thus took over the few existing hostels and training centres that existed in the early 1970s. There was, however, very little experience of learning disability in these new Social Services Departments, or in the previously small 'special needs' sections of Education Departments. When this is taken with the fact that there were also, for a brief period in the first half of the 1970s, substantial sources of capital finance, i.e. money to build buildings, it meant that Local Authorities looked to the DHSS for guidance, which came in the form of 'Building Notes'(see Dalgleish (1983) for implications of these 'environmental constraints').

There was thus a rapid expansion of standard 'models' for hostels, training centres and special schools representing the 'community care' end of the White Paper's plans. Summary figures from a consultative document published in 1976 show the number of residential care places in England in local authority, private and voluntary homes rising from 5,900 in 1969 to 9,500 in 1974 and the hospital population falling from 60,000 in 1969 to 55,000 in 1974 (DHSS 1976). Quite a lot of the new places were, however, filled by people moving into hostels from the family home, and quite a lot of the reduction in hospital places was due to a de facto halt in admission of children and the death of older patients. In many places hostels were seen as only for 'the cream', which did not include many in hospital. Given that the final targets of the White Paper were 33,700 community places and 33,000 hospital places by 1991, considerably faster rates of growth would be necessary. This was unlikely, given the effect on capital of the oil crisis of the mid-1970s, but also given a much stronger debate then taking place over responsibility for care and the appropriateness of various types of care. There was a substantial body of opinion, some from within the health service itself, for a unified service to supersede the roles currently undertaken by the social, education, and health services (Elliot 1972, 1975; Pilkington 1974). Observers of the Scandinavian scene, especially Sweden (Day 1974; Race and Race 1978), noted their status in the learning disability world as a result of such a move. Others, such as Gunzburg

(1973), did not go so far as proposing a new service, but stressed the importance of the 'multi-disciplinary team'. This approach, or variants of it, was to continue as an ideal for the next twenty-five years, and to be bedevilled by the relative status of team members (see Chapter 6).

Talk of change and movement for change – The Jay Committee and normalisation

The year 1975 saw not only the oil crisis mentioned above, but a significant starting point of a debate, at least in a much more public way than hitherto, about the place of the health service in the field of learning disability. As we have seen, the discussion about a unified service had some small weight in the even smaller area of academia and services that learning disability represented, but it took the Secretary of State at the DHSS, Barbara Castle, to try and carry on the work of her Labour predecessor, Richard Crossman, in changing the entrenched power of the medical model. She tackled the task in typically combative style. In a speech to the National Society in February 1975, she set up three initiatives which had a major impact on changing ideas, though it would take other developments, as we shall see, to begin real changes in practice.

Mrs Castle's initiatives were, first, the setting up of a 'National Development Group (NDG) for the Mentally Handicapped' under the chairmanship of Professor Peter Mittler to 'play an active part in the development of policy at the DHSS' (Cunningham 1975). Together with the NDG, which would act at the central level of the DHSS, was set up a National Development Team (NDT) whose job it would be to go round to Local Authorities and health areas, advising on the implementation of DHSS policies. Second, Mrs Castle announced the setting up of a Committee of Inquiry into Mental Handicap Nursing and Care, under Mrs Peggy Jay. The importance of these first two initiatives in the debates which followed has tended to overshadow the third initiative, whereby Mrs Castle set in train a 'reorganisation of the medical role in mental handicap'. Perhaps another reason why this third initiative is little discussed is that, apart from appointing consultants to Area Health Authorities rather than special hospitals, their position remained largely unchanged by the 'reorganisation'. Importantly, this included their power over admission and discharge; their 'clinical autonomy'.

As for the other initiatives, political events and the restriction on public spending in the years between 1975 and 1979 make it hard to assess the real impact of the NDG and NDT, and it took until 1979 for the Jay Committee report to be published. Certainly the NDG was active in publication, producing pamphlets on a number of topics (NDG 1977a; 1977b; 1977c; 1977d). 'Pamphlet 5', on day services, was the most widely used document and, given the furore it raised by setting out a 'model' of the 'Social Education Centre', the most controversial (see Chapters 3 and 5). In practice, however, with evidence to the Jay Committee still revealing the powerful interests within the services at odds with one another (e.g. Kushlick *et al*. 1976) it is perhaps inevitable that the NDG, a group whose membership seems to have been designed to 'balance' the views of the medical, nursing and other professions, should have produced compromises. In particular, though its final two reports (NDG 1978, 1980) produced far more in terms of recommendations about standards, they did so within the status quo of services, i.e. on the assumption that residential care would largely be provided in hospitals and hostels, schooling in special schools and daytime activity for adults in large adult training centres. The balance of power within the DHSS, which Barbara Castle had attempted to by-pass with this 'independent' group, still seems to have been retained by the civil servants, and thus advice to ministers in the incoming Conservative government of 1979 appears to have looked to maintain the status quo. Further evidence for this is suggested by the fact that the NDG was wound up in the early 1980s, whereas the NDT, headed until 1986 by a psychiatrist, continues, and also by the reaction and subsequent inaction that followed the report of the Jay Committee in 1979.

As that report was published, of course, there was also the most radical change of government ideology for many years, with Mrs Thatcher's incoming Conservative administration heralding a period that was to alter drastically the lives of many people. Such was the impact of those eighteen years that it is often forgotten that in its beginnings the new government did a number of 'deals' with the still strong unions, before going on later to legislate and publicly berate them into impotence. One such deal appears to have been their reaction to the Jay Committee report, though many other factors, not least the dead hand of the DHSS, conspired to dismiss what was, in its way, the most radical set of proposals that the learning disability field had seen.

As well as its origins in the debates we have described above, the Jay Committee was sitting at the same time as the emergence of two further developments, one from within services, one from a small but influential group of academics and other activists. The first was a number of attempts from the service system to facilitate and encourage joint working between services, most notably Health and Social Services Departments. What first became known as 'joint financing', accompanied by the setting up of 'joint planning teams' at local level, was followed by a number of financial carrots being dangled in front of Social Services Departments to take people out of hospital, and then by schemes to prevent people from going into hospital in the first place. The problems with such efforts were, first, that the money for these schemes only represented a fraction of the total expenditure on learning disability services, and second, whether such joint working could be carried out successfully by two bodies with entirely different structures, entirely different political control (elected councillors for social services and appointed health authority members) and, very often, different geographical boundaries. The effect of these schemes by the time Jay reported was therefore small, and lent further weight to those advocating a joint service.

The second aspect relevant to Jay's findings was the impact of the developing concept of normalisation. As we shall detail in Chapter 12, and have noted briefly above, this idea, as coined in Scandinavia in the 1960s had had an influence on those groups critical of the medical model of care. As developed by Wolfensberger and others in the 1972 publication of the same name, normalisation began to be viewed as having wider implications. The analysis formed the backbone of campaigning by various groups in the late 1970s, notably Campaign for the Mentally Handicapped (CMH) (O'Brien and Tyne 1981), and, through the influence of certain key members of the Jay Committee had a direct effect on the 'Model of Care' proposed by that committee.

The brief of the committee, as well as that implied by its title, was to address a specific recommendation in an earlier committee, the Briggs Committee (DHSS *et al.*, 1972) that a separate profession be set up for the care of people with learning difficulties. In interpreting this brief, the Jay Committee chose to propose a 'model of care' based on the following broad principles:

a) Mentally handicapped people have a right to enjoy normal patterns of life within the community.
b) Mentally handicapped people have a right to be treated as individuals.
c) Mentally handicapped people will require additional help from the communities in which they live and from professional services if they are to develop to their maximum potential as individuals.

(Jay Committee Report 1979: 35)

The influence of normalisation is clear, especially as developed by Wolfensberger into a 'model' service in Nebraska (Wolfensberger 1975) which was visited by at least one member of the Jay Committee, and given substance in the evaluation instrument called Program Analysis of Service Systems (PASS) (Wolfensberger and Glenn 1975), which looks not just at the interactions and activities of service users, but the environmental and organisational setting, and the images conveyed of the people involved. Its influence on the Jay Committee is further evidenced by their 'Service Principles' which follow the broad principles above:

a) Mentally handicapped people should use normal services wherever possible.
b) Existing networks of community support should be strengthened by professional services rather than supplanted by them.
c) 'Specialised' services or organisations for mentally handicapped people should be provided only to the extent that they demonstrably meet or are likely to meet additional needs that cannot be met by the general services.
d) If we are to meet the many and diverse needs of mentally handicapped people we need maximum co-ordination of services both within and between services and at all levels. The concept of a life plan seems essential if co-ordination and continuity of care is to be achieved.
e) Finally, if we are to establish and maintain high quality services for a group of people who cannot easily articulate and press their just claims, we need someone to intercede on behalf of mentally handicapped people in obtaining services.

(Jay Committee Report 1979: 36–37)

A glance at the *Valuing People* White Paper (DoH 2001) reveals an amazing number of similarities with the above principles, from ideas of lifestyle planning, through joint working to social inclusion. The fact that the White Paper is presented as a 'New Strategy' also shows how successful was the resistance and eventual burial of the Jay Committee Report and, as we shall see, the lack of attribution of current thinking to the ideas of normalisation. The Jay Committee Report probably represented the most public acceptance of a change in attitude within the broad field of learning disability, and together with *An Ordinary Life*, a proposal for a comprehensive model of residential care based on ordinary housing, which appeared a year later (King's Fund 1980), the most public challenge to the still medically dominated service. Even within the Jay Report, however, notes of dissent from some members, especially the minority report by D.O. Williams, Chairman of the staff side of the Whitley Council for the Health Services (essentially the negotiating body for nurses' terms of service), demonstrated the tremendous professional and employment issues at stake. With the incoming government, as noted above, anxious to buy time in its dealings with the unions, especially those with public sympathy such as the nursing unions, and also to trim public spending to carry out its commitment to tax cuts, the prospect of a protracted battle that might hand over more power to local authority services was not great. So, as Ryan notes, by 1981 'The Jay report . . . a ground breaking inquiry . . . had been quietly buried and with it the heated controversy and commitment to extra expenditure that the government was too anxious to avoid' (Ryan and Thomas 1987: 153).

As for normalisation, the next decade was to see its adoption and adaptation, sometimes to the point of unrecognisability, whilst at the same time much bigger forces were determining the fate of services.

Money talks – the NHS and Community Care Act and after

The 1970s had therefore seen a plethora of debates and discussions on the hospital/community issue and launched, in normalisation and the ideas around it, what Tyne (1987) was later to describe as a 'social movement'. That this was initiated by a small group of people, led by Tyne and Williams' training organisation, Community and Mental Handicap Education and Research Association (CMHERA), then growing into a national network of people attempting to implement change, may be a tribute to the power of the ideas, but it also reveals the fragility of such movements. The government, having buried the Jay report, issued a 'consultative document' in 1981 which, whilst it 're-emphasises' a commitment to community care, only mandated a hospital closure programme, and that in very vague terms (DHSS 1981). Alternatives to both hospital and the predominant local form of residential care, the hostel, were not seriously put forward.

Developments in classification of people illustrate the picture still more. In a report in 1978, which assumed some currency for a while, the NDT, described above, divided 'mentally handicapped people' in hospitals into four categories, based around their continence, ambulence and behaviour. These were then linked to recommended sorts of service with only the 'best' group considered suitable for immediate discharge to 'home or hostel' though some of this group 'may be appropriately placed in group homes'. As for the others, various periods of time in 'training units' is suggested before 'care in the community' can be granted, and even this will be largely in hostels. As with all other classifications, the description is related to behaviour, and the 'needs' to existing resources, rather than the 'ordinary life' of the Jay Committee and the normalisation movement.

Meanwhile, as the Thatcher government got into full cost-cutting stride, it faced an interesting paradox. On the one hand, expensive long-stay hospitals on valuable land were being criticised by the normalisation movement and others, thus suggesting hospital closure as a profitable way to meet the demands of the field. At the same time, however, Thatcher's political project to run down the power of Local Authorities (Cutler and Waine 1997) was at odds with a hospital closure programme that would increase the alternative, Local Authority, services. The Local Authorities, for their part, saw the expense of their long-stay institutions mounting, at a time of cuts in goverment financial support, yet the alternatives, especially in residential care in ordinary housing, appeared even more expensive. Thus while there began to appear some nationally known 'ordinary housing' projects, these were rare, and usually needed a voluntary agency, such as Barnardo's in The North West of England, to be prepared to 'experiment' (Alaszewski 1986). Similarly, despite a follow on report from the Kings Fund (1984) on daytime activity, which advocated more effort in finding real employment for people, such schemes were rare, especially as unemployment nationally was escalating. As we shall discuss in more detail in Chapter 6, the 1980s also saw a rapid growth, encouraged by the government, in residential care being provided by private and voluntary agencies. This was especially true in homes for elderly people, which had a tradition of such care as a significant part of provision already, but the notion expanded into learning disability services. For example, Mencap, the name now used by the former National Society, set up a parallel 'Homes Foundation' which started to open many 'ordinary houses', though initially these tended to be large houses of ten to twelve beds with very strict admission criteria. Other examples were private 'community' projects, often set up by groups of nurses from the closing hospitals.

Faced with the extra social security payments that were used for places in private care, the Government looked to the Audit Commission to try and deal with its mounting bill. Again, more detail of this process is given in Chapter 6, but the effects on services began to be felt in arrangements to close hospitals, and the beginnings of a wider range of alternatives. The coincidence of these primarily economic moves and the growth of the normalisation movement, tended to result in the gradual introduction of a standard 'model' for residential care in terms of the four- to six-bedded 'ordinary house', though in terms of daytime provision the lack of commercial prospects of training centres meant that they were less subject to alternative agencies to the Local Authority. Residential care was also provided by some health authorities in ordinary housing, and here too, normalisation, or a certain version of it, became part of nurse training.

The bigger picture then again had its impact on services, in that, following the report of Sir Roy Griffiths (DoH 1988) and a government response in the form of a White Paper (DoH 1989), the final working out of the impact of growing social security spending and the growing private sector came in the NHS and Community Care Act of 1990 and subsequent guidance (Hudson 1994). As will be discussed in Chapter 6, however, the effect of this Act was more in terms of organisational change than on the sort of services provided. The hospitals continued to close, the independent sector took up more and more of the provision of services, and the system began more and more to resemble the situation in the USA. There, the massive de-institutionalisation of the 1970s, again partially influenced by normalisation, when combined with an existing market system of welfare, produced a vast range of services, some extremely radical, some extremely institutional, with little coherent pattern observable (Schwartz 1997). The diffusion of services also had the effect of diluting the effect of normalisation in the USA. In the UK the dilution was compounded by academic criticism of normalisation, and considerable confusion over the differences between it and Wolfensberger's reformulation and development of the theory of 'Social Role Valorization' (1983). That story is elaborated in Chapter 11, but in terms of its effects on services, the following factors were to take effect: a reduction of the 'movement' into factional disputes; the growing power of the disability movement for self-determination and rights; and the fragmented nature of service provision in the 1990s. This meant that never again was a single set of ideas to have the same impact.

Equally fragmented, as the 1990s wore on, was the issue of classification, and in view of the thesis of this chapter that services have tended to reflect the image of people brought about by classification, it would be expected, as was the case, that debates and arguments would still rage about classification, given the fragmented nature of current services. On the one side, with the increasing move for self-determination and rights, allies of people with learning difficulties have sought to discover what they would wish to be called. This task is, of course, extremely difficult, given arguments over whether any one subset of a group can represent the group as a whole, and whether the group wishes to be identified by any label at all, but those who have attempted to ascertain people's views tend to use the term 'learning difficulties'. From the service system has come the term 'learning disability'. According to the Centre for Research and Information into Mental Disability (CRIMD) (1992) the term was 'introduced by the Department of Health in 1991 to replace "mental handicap"' and it certainly appeared 'officially' in DoH guidance following the NHS and Community Care Act (DOHSSI 1991).

As with its reaction to normalisation, the UK seems to differ in this regard from most of the rest of the English speaking world, where neither term seems to be used, and further complication occurs when the term learning difficulties is taken to mean different things in the educational world than in other parts of the service system. Given the power of the Department of Health in this field, and especially when Mencap adopted the term (despite many arguments at local societies, who tended to prefer 'mental handicap'), 'learning disability' appears to have achieved dominance, though, as we explain in the Introduction to this book, there are still powerful reasons for challenging that. The passion seems to have reduced somewhat in this debate, however, perhaps because there may now be the possibility of some development in services, whereas the argument often seemed to take energy away from pushing for those developments.

Moving into the millennium – services in need of a strategy

We are now at the point in our history of services where current patterns, or more accurately the lack of a pattern, became established. From the easily describable range of services that held sway, even into the early 1990s, has emerged a veritable supermarket of service modes, though as *Facing the Facts* and *Valuing People* observe, this contains many services that display practices and other attributes that would have been expected to have disappeared by now, had the rhetoric become reality. Two other issues, however, need to be mentioned, since they have come to prominence in the late 1980s and through the 1990s. Though not strictly about service 'forms', they have had some influence on the development of services and certainly appear to have resulted in a much greater public debate on learning disability issues.

One, alluded to above, is the growth of advocacy, and more broadly of self-determination and rights as the means by which oppressed groups have sought to redress the power that society, and society's representatives in the service system, have held over them. The ideas of advocacy were in full swing in the 1980s, though initially rather more sizeable in literature than in practice, and even had legislation in the form of the Disabled Persons (Services Consultation and Representation) Act of 1986. This Act, however, pushed through by Labour MP Tom Clarke in a rare success for a Private Members Bill, was never fully implemented, and was swallowed up by the NHS and Community Care Act of 1990. It was not until the growing power of the disability lobby in the 1990s, backed up by academic theory in the form of the social model of disability, began to gain some concessions from the government, that a broader possibility for people with learning difficulties to be considered one of the groups who needed to be involved in decisions became more acceptable. More of the discussion on these issues is found in Chapter 10, but in terms of the effects of advocacy, and especially self-advocacy, many public statements have been made affirming the rights of people to be involved in decisions, not only about their own lives, but also as part of strategic planning for learning disability services. This includes the *Valuing People* White Paper. Mencap changed their constitution in 1999, to allow representation of people with learning difficulties in their management structures, and planning mechanisms, especially since the 'modernising agenda' of the New Labour government, elected in 1997, has included specific demands for representation and consultation. Some have been critical, however, e.g. Walmsley and Downer (1997), of the slow pace of involvement of people with learning difficulties as opposed to other groups, and others still see the involvement and consultation as lacking any real power, even with the 'stronger' groups. The Disability Discrimination Act of 1995 and the Direct Payments Act of 1999 represent the legislative result of this movement, and it also sets the scene for people to take advantage of the Human Rights Act (1998) which came into effect in October 2000. It remains to be seen, however, whether these widespread 'rights' will result in real change to services, and whether the much trumpeted involvement of people with learning difficulties in the development and implementation of the *Valuing People* White Paper will have had the desired effect.

Doubts on this score come from reflection on the other key issue that has been part of the growing public debate on learning disability issues, though again much more detailed discussion is found elsewhere, especially in Chapter 13. This is the debate around all the aspects of what has come to be called the 'quality of life.' As we noted in relation to Tredgold's comments in the early 1950s, and the German *euthanasie* policy of the 1930s and 1940s, modern critics of such views need to make the connection with current debates on genetic screening, embryology, and the still existing provisions of the Abortion (Amendment) Act of 1992. The views, on the one hand, of the disability movement, especially disabled women, on the image of disabled people that current practices represent, and the ever-increasing utilitarian position revealed by the growth of genetic research seem to be poles apart. Cases of people with learning difficulties being denied medical treatment have been known within the field for many years, but received an unexpected airing in late 2000 when the winner of the highly popular television series *Big Brother* donated his prize to a young woman with Down's syndrome to enable her to go to the USA for heart treatment denied her in the UK. Public views in reaction were strongly in favour of the woman, but, like the show itself, quickly became yesterday's news.

This history of services and classification therefore ends with the observation of a divided, in fact not just divided but fragmented, picture. In true postmodern fashion, the big debates of the 1970s, 1980s and early 1990s between normalisation and the institutional system, between the domination of the medical model and a social approach, and between the rights to self-determination of oppressed groups and a professionalised service system seem to have diffused into a pragmatic task-oriented approach to services. Planning and strategy seems to be overwhelmed by the everyday pressures of survival in a welfare system which still resembles a marketplace, despite the 'modernising' efforts of the New Labour government. Organisational change is again in the offing, with 'care trusts' likely to take over more services for adults, and the training of staff in learning disabilities, despite the welcome objective in the White Paper for a standard qualification, still likely to take its customary place as a small, under-resourced part of new qualifications in health and social welfare.

Visiting services to observe students on placement, or as part of the few remaining PASSING workshops to teach people about 'Social Role Valorization'

(Wolfensberger and Thomas 1983; Race 1999), I am struck by how many of the themes covered by the thesis cited at the beginning of this chapter still remain. Congregation, segregation and devaluation even in the midst of community life all remain. Public fear of the 'otherness' of learning disability, stoked up further by a public media that seems unable to take a broad view on any issue, has left people in probably as vulnerable a position as thirty years ago when the scene was dominated by the institutions. In keeping with the development of a society where, as a radio news item reported in one of the many 'focus on the new millennium' surveys, primary school children's ambitions were centred more on winning the lottery than on anything they might achieve by their own efforts, the fate of people with learning difficulties, and the services they might receive, seems more and more dependent on their postcode, and the attitudes and organisations that locality contains.

References

Acts of Parliament

Poor Law Amendment Act (1834) 4 and 5 Will IV, C76
Lunatic Asylums Act (1853) London, HMSO
Idiots Act (1886) London, HMSO
Mental Deficiency Act (1913) London, HMSO
Education Act (1944) London, HMSO
Mental Health Act (1959) London, HMSO
Education (Handicapped Children) Act (1970) London, HMSO
Disabled Persons (Services Consultation and Representation) Act (1986), London, HMSO
National Health Service and Community Care Act (1990), London, HMSO
Abortion (Amendment) Act (1992), London, HMSO
Disability Discrimination Act (1995), London, HMSO
Direct Payments Act (1999) London, The Stationery Office
Human Rights Act (1998) London, The Stationery Office

General references

Alaszewski, A. (1986) *Institutional Care and the Mentally Handicapped*, London, Croom Helm.
Annas, G.J. (ed) (1992) *The Nazi Doctors and the Nuremburg Code: Human Rights in Human Experimentation*, New York/Oxford, Oxford University Press.
Baller, W.R., Charles, D.C. and Miller, E.L. (1967) Midlife attainment of the mentally retarded – a longitudinal study, *Gen. Psychol. Mon.* 75: 235–329.
Baranjay, E.P. (1971) *The Mentally Handicapped Adolescent*, Oxford, Pergamon.
Barnes, M. (1997) Families and empowerment. In: P. Ramcharan, G. Roberts, G. Grant and J. Borland (eds) *Empowerment in Everyday Life: Learning Disability*, London, Jessica Kingsley.
Binding, K. and Hoche, A. (1920) *The Release of the Destruction of Life Devoid of Value*, Leipzig, F. Meiner.

Campaign for the Mentally Handicapped (1971) *The White Paper and Future Services for the Mentally Handicapped*, London, CMH Publications.

Campaign for the Mentally Handicapped (1972) *Even Better Services for the Mentally Handicapped*, London, CMH Publications.

Castell, J.H.F. and Mittler, P.J. (1965) Intelligence of patients in subnormality hospitals: a survey of admissions in 1961, *Brit. J. Psychiat*, 111: 219–225.

Centre for Research and Information into Mental Disability (1992) *Healthcare for People with a Learning Disability – a Discussion Document*, Department of Psychiatry, University of Birmingham.

Claridge, G.S. (1961) The Senior Occupation Centre and the practical application of research to the training of the severely subnormal, *Brit. J. Ment. Subn.*, 8: 11–16.

Clarke, A.D.B. and Blakemore, C.B. (1961) Age and perpetual motor transfer in imbeciles, *Brit. J. Psychol.*, 52, 125–131

Clarke, A.D.B. and Clarke, A.M. (1953) How constant is the IQ? *Lancet*, 2: 877.

Clarke, A.D.B. and Clarke, A.M. (1954) Cognitive changes in the feebleminded, *Brit. J. Psychol.*, 45: 173–179.

Clarke, A.D.B., Clarke, A.M. and Reiman, S. (1958) Cognitive and social changes in the feebleminded – three further studies, *Brit. J. Psychol*, 53: 321–330.

Crossman, R. (1977) *The Diaries of a Cabinet Minister Vol 3*, London, Hamish Hamilton.

Cunningham, J. (1975) Barbara and her begging bowl, *New Psychiatry*, 13 March: 4–7.

Cutler, T. and Waine, B. (1997) *Managing the Welfare State*, Oxford, Berg.

Dalgleish, M. (1983) Environmental constraints on residential services for mentally handicapped people: some findings from the Sheffield Development Project, *Mental Handicap*, 11: 102–105.

Day, K. (1974) Follow the Northern Lights, *New Psychiatry*, 28 November: 8–11.

Department of Health (1988) *Community Care: Agenda for Action (The Griffiths Report)*, London, HMSO.

Department of Health (1989) *Caring for People – Community Care in the Next Decade and Beyond*, Command 849, London, HMSO.

Department of Health (1999) *Facing the Facts: Services for People with Learning Disabilities. A Policy Impact Study of Social Care and Health Services*, London, The Stationery Office.

Department of Health (2001) *Valuing People – a New Strategy for Learning Disability for the 21st Century*, London, The Stationery Office.

Department of Health Social Service Inspectorate (1991) *Care Management and Assessment: Summary of Practice Guidance*, London, HMSO.

Department of Health and Social Security (1971) *Better Services for the Mentally Handicapped*. Command 4683, London, HMSO.

Department of Health and Social Security (1976) *Priorities in the Health and Social Services in England – a Consultative Document*, London, HMSO.

Department of Health and Social Security (1981) *Care in the Community – A Consultative Document on Moving Resources for Care in England*, London, HMSO.

Department of Health and Social Security, Scottish Home and Health Department and Welsh Office (1972) *Report of the Committee on Nursing (The Briggs Report)*, London, HMSO.

Elliot, J. (1972) Eight propositions for mental handicap, *Brit. J. Ment. Subn.*, 9: Pt 1.

Elliot, J. (1975) Segregated ghetto or better services?, *Res. Soc. Work.*, 15: 4–5.

Goffman, E. (1961) *Asylums – Essays on the Social Situation of Mental Patients and Other Inmates*, Gordon City, NY, Doubleday.

Gunzburg, H.C. (1957) Therapy and social training for the feebleminded youth, *Brit. J. Med. Psychol.*, 30: 42–48.

Gunzburg, H.C. (1961) The case for comprehensive training, *Brit. J. Ment. Subn.*, 7: 53–61.

Gunzburg, H.C. (1973) The role of the psychologist in manipulating the institutional environment. In: A.D.B. Clarke and A.M. Clarke (eds). *Mental Retardation and Behavioural Research: IRMR Study Group No 4*, London, Churchill Livingstone.

Hilliard, L.T. and Kirman, B.H. (1965) *Mental Deficiency*, London, Churchill.

Home Office, Department of Education and Science, Ministry of Housing and Local Government, Ministry of Health (1968) *Report of the Committee on Local Authority and Allied Personal Social Services (The Seebohm Report)*, Command 3703, London, HMSO.

Howe Report (1969) *Report of the Committee of Enquiry into Allegations of Ill Treatment of Patients and Others at the Ely Hospital, Cardiff*, Command 3795, London, HMSO.

Hudson, R. (1994) Management and Finance. In N. Malin (ed.) *Implementing Community Care*, Buckingham, Open University Press.

Itard, J.M.G. (1801) *The Wild Boy of Aveyron*, Trans. G.M. Humphrey (1932) New York, New York Press.

Jay Committee (1979) *Report of the Committee of Inquiry into Mental Handicap Nursing and Care*, Command 7468, London, HMSO.

Jones, K., Brown, J. and Bradshaw, J. (1979) *Issues in Social Policy*, London, Routledge and Kegan Paul.

King, R.D. and Raynes, N.V. (1968) An operational measure of inmate management in residential institutions, *Soc. Sci. Med.*, 2: 41–53.

King, R.D., Raynes, N.V. and Tizard, J. (1971) *Patterns of Residential Care: Sociological Studies in Institutions for Handicapped Children*, London, Routledge and Kegan Paul.

King's Fund (1980) *An Ordinary Life – Comprehensive Locally Based Services for Mentally Handicapped People*. London, King's Fund Centre.

King's Fund (1984) *An Ordinary Working Life – Vocational Services for People with Mental Handicaps*. Kings Fund Project Paper No. 50, London, King's Fund Centre.

Kirk, S.A. (1958) *Early Education of the Mentally Retarded*, Chicago, University of Chicago Press.

Kushlick, A., Felce, D., Palmer, J. and Smith, J. (1976) *Evidence to the Committee of Inquiry into Mental Handicap Nursing and Care from the Health Care Evaluation Research Team*, Winchester, HCERT.

Lifton, R.J. (1986) *The Nazi Doctors: Medically Killing and Psychology of Genocide*, New York, Basic Books.

Locke, J. (1689) *An Essay Concerning Human Understanding*, London, Basset.

Martin, J. (1984) *Hospitals in Trouble*, Oxford, Basil Blackwell.

Matthews, F.B. (1954) *Mental Health Services*, London, Shaw.

Ministry of Health (1962) *A Hospital Plan for England and Wales*, London, HMSO.

Ministry of Health (1963) *Health and Welfare: the Development of Community Care*, London, HMSO.

Moorman, C. (1967) A social education centre, *Brit. J. Ment. Subn.* 13: 88–92.

Morris, J. (1991) *Pride Against Prejudice: Transforming Attitudes to Disability*, London, The Women's Press.

Morris, P. (1969) *Put Away: A Sociological Study of Institutions for the Mentally Retarded*, London, Routledge and Kegan Paul.

National Development Group for the Mentally Handicapped (NDG) (1977a) *Pamphlet No. 2 – Mentally Handicapped Children: A Plan for Action*, London, HMSO.

National Development Group for the Mentally Handicapped (NDG) (1977b) *Pamphlet No. 3 – Helping Mentally Handicapped School Leavers*, London, HMSO.

National Development Group for the Mentally Handicapped (NDG) (1977c) *Pamphlet No. 4 – Residential Short-Term Care for Mentally Handicapped People: Suggestions for Action*, London, HMSO.

National Development Group for the Mentally Handicapped (NDG) (1977d) *Pamphlet No. 5 – Day Services for Mentally Handicapped Adults*, London, HMSO.

National Development Group for the Mentally Handicapped (NDG) (1978) *Helping Mentally Handicapped People in Hospital: A Report to the Secretary of State for Social Services*, London, HMSO.

National Development Group for the Mentally Handicapped (NDG) (1980) *Improving the Quality of Services for Mentally Handicapped People – A Checklist of Standards*, London, HMSO.

National Development Team for the Mentally Handicapped (NDT) (1978) *First Report 1976–77*, London, HMSO.

National Society for Mentally Handicapped Children (1974) The stress of having a subnormal child. In: D.M. Boswell and J.M. Wingrove (eds), *The Handicapped Person in the Community*, London, Tavistock (in association with Open University Press).

Nihara, K., Foster, R., Shellhaus, M. and Leland, H. (1969) *Adaptive Behaviour Scale 1st edition*, Washington, DC, AAMD.

O'Brien, J. and Tyne, A. (1981) *Normalisation: A Foundation for Effective Services*, London, CMH Publications.

O'Connor, N. (1965) The successful employment of the mentally handicapped, In: L.T. Hilliard and B.H. Kirman (eds), *Mental Deficiency*, London, Churchill.

O'Connor, N. and Tizard, J. (1954) A survey of patients in twelve mental deficiency institutions, *Brit. Med. J.*, I: 16–20.

Oliver, M. (1990) *The Politics of Disablement*, London, Macmillan.

Owen, D. (1965) *English Philanthropy 1660–1960*, London, Oxford University Press.

Pearson, K. and Jaederholm, G.A. (1914) *On the Continuity of Mental Defect: Questions of the Day and of the Fray. No. VIII Mendelism and the Problems of Mental Defect*, Dept of Applied Statistics, University College London.

Pilkington T.L. (1974) *Patterns of Care for the Mentally Retarded in the United Kingdom*. Mental Handicap Bulletin No. 14, London, King's Fund Centre.

Price, I.J. (1967) The industrial training and social education of subnormal adults, *Brit. J. Ment. Subn.*, 10, 113–117.

Race, D.G. (1977) *Investigation into the Effects of Different Caring Environments on the Social Competence of Mentally Handicapped Adults*, Unpublished PhD thesis – University of Reading.

Race, D.G. (1999) *Social Role Valorization and the English Experience*, Wilding and Birch, London.

Race, D.G. and Race D.M. (1978) Services for the mentally handicapped in Sweden, *Child, Health Care and Development*, 4(1): 12–17.

Raynes, N.V. and King, R.D. (1968) *The Measurement of Child Management in Institutions for the Retarded*. Proc. First. Cong. Int. Assoc. Sci. Study. Ment. Def., Baltimore, University Park Press.

Royal Medico-Psychological Association (1971) RMPA memorandum on future patterns of care of the mentally subnormal, *Brit. J. Psychiat.*, 2: 119–20.

Ryan, J. and Thomas, F. (1987) *The Politics of Mental Handicap*, 2nd edition, Harmondsworth, Penguin.

Schwartz, D.B. (1997) *Who Cares – Rediscovering Community*, Oxford, Westview Press.

Sullivan, M (1992) *The Politics of Social Policy*, Hemel Hempstead, Harvester Wheatsheaf.

Tawney, R. (1938) *Religion and the Rise of Capitalism: a Historical study; with a Prefatory Note by Charles Gore*, Harmondsworth, Penguin.

Thane, P. (1982) *The Foundations of the Welfare State*, London, Longman.

Tizard, J. (1958) Introduction. In A.M. Clarke and A.D.B. Clarke (eds) *Mental Deficiency – The Changing Outlook,* 1st edition, London, Methuen.

Tizard, J. (1964) *Community Services for the Mentally Handicapped*, London, Oxford University Press.

Tredgold, A.F. (1909) The Feebleminded – a social danger, *Eugenics Review*, 1: 97–104.

Tredgold, A.F. (1922) *Mental Deficiency (Amentia)*, 4th edition, London, Baillière Tindall & Cox.

Tredgold, A.F. (1952) *A Textbook on Mental Deficiency (Amentia)*, 8th edition, London, Ballière, Tindall & Cox.

Tyne, A. (1987) Shaping Community Services: the impact of an idea. In: N. Malin (ed.) *Reassessing Community Care*, London, Croom Helm.

Walmsley, J. and Downer, J. (1997) Shouting the loudest: self-advocacy, power and diversity. In: P. Ramcharan, G. Roberts, G. Grant and J. Borland (eds) *Empowerment in Everyday Life: Learning Disability*, London, Jessica Kingsley.

Williams, P. (1967) Industrial training and remunerative employment of the profoundly retarded, *Brit.J. Ment. Subn.*, 13(1).

Wolfensberger, W. (1972) *The Principle of Normalization in Human Services*, Toronto, NIMR.

Wolfensberger, W. (1975) The Principle of Normalization as it applies to services for the severely handicapped. In: H. Mallik, S. Uspeh and J. Muller (eds) *Comprehensive Vocational Rehabilitation Services for Severely Disabled Persons*, Washington, DC, George Washington University.

Wolfensberger, W. (1983) Social Role Valorization: A proposed new term for the Principle of Normalization. *Mental Retardation*, 21: 234–239.

Wolfensberger, W. (2000) *Historical Expressions of Learning Disability in Language and Art – Implications for Our Times*. Presentation made at University of Newcastle, July 2000.

Wolfensberger, W. and Glenn, L. (1975) *Program Analysis of Service Systems (PASS),* 3rd edition, Field Manual, Toronto, NIMR.

Wolfensberger, W. and Thomas, S. (1983) *Program Analysis of Service System's Implementation of Normalization Goals (PASSING)* 2nd edition, Toronto, NIMR.

Wood Report (1929) *Report of the Mental Deficiency Committee*, London, HMSO.

Chapter 3

Residential and day services for adults

Paul Williams

Introduction

In an earlier chapter for a similar book to this (Williams 1995a), I reviewed the evidence from research and official sources relating to residential and day care for people with learning difficulties in Britain in the mid-1990s. I will present an updated summary here before embarking on a rather different approach to considering these services.

The White Paper *Valuing People* (Department of Health 2001) estimates that there are about 63,000 adults with learning difficulties in residential care in England. The total number of adults with severe learning difficulties is estimated as 145,000; the majority are likely to be living at home with their families. There are about 56,000 places in social services day provision, and some opportunities available in supported work or in further education. A substantial number of adults receive no day provision outside their place of residence (the White Paper states that at least 20,000 people with severe learning difficulties do not attend a day service). Since the NHS and Community Care Act 1990 there has been a great increase in the number of residential services provided by voluntary and private agencies; this has been far less the case with day provision, the majority of which is still provided directly by local social services departments. In the past decade there has been a large expansion of residential provision in the form of small housing in ordinary community settings, though substantial numbers of people still live in larger hostels, hospital units or 'village communities'. One of the concerns of the White Paper is wide variability of both quantity and quality of provision across the country (Department of Health 1999).

By and large, community care for people with learning difficulties has been a great success. Because of the relatively small numbers of people involved, standards have been able to reflect high values – for example, that people should live in small numbers in ordinary housing in order to maximise homely experiences and opportunities for inclusion in local community life. Such standards have not been applied in services for other groups, for example older people.

Research into different living arrangements has not produced any real surprises. Some people like living alone, with whatever support they need, but there is a risk of loneliness and isolation (Flynn 1989). Placement of adults with families can work well, but there are difficulties in finding suitable families (Dagnan and Drewett 1988). Living in lodgings has a mixed reputation: there have been stories of people being turned out during the day, for example, amidst other stories of great dedication and commitment by individual landlords or landladies (Ferrity *et al*. 1986). Some health authorities and social services departments are still stuck with large-scale hostel-type accommodation widely regarded as unsatisfactory (Heron 1982). There are some well-known 'village communities', such as Botton village in Yorkshire and Ravenswood in Berkshire, providing self-contained care for a large number of people on one site, usually in a rural setting (see Segal 1990). While the quality of care in large establishments can be good, the problem is the severe constraint put on social inclusion in ordinary community life (Lynn 2001). Indeed, a strong message can be sent out by such services that people with learning difficulties must be socially excluded because of the 'nuisance' they present in ordinary society (Wolfensberger 1998; Race 1999).

One idea that has gained ground in the 1990s is that of 'supported living'. The housing arrangements for people with learning difficulties are separated from the requirement for supportive care. This opens up possibilities that people may purchase and manage their own care, with whatever help they need, through schemes of direct payment, though this development is in its infancy (Holman and Bewley 1999). Probably in the future we will see more possibilities for people to own or rent their own homes, with care and support being provided and funded separately. This will give people greater security of accommodation, and will reduce the risk of agencies and support workers seeing themselves as owners and controllers of accommodation, rather than as guests and servants in the homes of the people with learning difficulties themselves. The White Paper (Department of Health 2001) introduces a policy and funding framework called 'Supporting People', to be implemented in April 2003, which will 'bring together resources from several existing programmes into a new grant to local authorities which can be applied more flexibly to fund support services for people . . . wherever they live' (p. 74).

Most studies of accommodation of people in small numbers in ordinary houses in ordinary community settings have shown positive outcomes in terms both of quality of experiences and of personal development (Emerson *et al*. 1999). There is some evidence that Social Role Valorisation (SRV – see Chapter 11 in this book; Wolfensberger 1998; Race 1999; Williams 2001) is best achieved by 'life-sharing' arrangements where people with learning difficulties and non-disabled people share accommodation and activities on an equal basis (Williams 1995c; see also the description of L'Arche philosophy later in this chapter).

Day services provide a wide range of different functions, and the national scene is as chaotic as it has ever been. Many services still suffer from trying to implement aims that are not compatible with the size and location of their buildings inherited from earlier times. New initiatives, such as the King's Fund 'Changing Days' project (McIntosh and Whittaker 1998), struggle to impact on large, outdated provision. The concept of 'model coherency' (see Chapter 7 in this book) would suggest that the future should lie in a separation of functions of day services, so that leisure and social facilities can develop and be managed separately from therapeutic services, therapy separately from education, and education separately from employment support. The large range of often incompatible aims that many current day services are expected to meet has been well described by Carter (1981). The White Paper (Department of Health 2001) outlines a five-year programme to modernise day services, but the issue of 'model coherency' remains unaddressed and the confused global concept of the 'day service' remains.

The history of residential care

David Race has outlined the general history of services for people with learning difficulties in Chapter 2. It is worth recounting here, though, how concepts of residential care have changed over the last 150 years. Ironically, recent concepts have come full circle from those held in the mid-nineteenth century. Samuel Howe, an American pioneer of services for disabled people, was invited to open a new residence for blind people in 1866. He used the opportunity to criticise the establishment of large institutions. He said that the only buildings that should be specially built are 'school rooms, recreation rooms, recitation rooms, music rooms and workshops; and these should be in or near the centre of a dense population. For other purposes, ordinary houses would suffice' (Wolfensberger 1975).

Dr John Langdon Down, who gave the first systematic description of Down's syndrome, which is named after him, was superintendent of the first large residential establishment in Britain for people with learning difficulties – Earlswood Asylum in Surrey – for ten years until 1868 when he left to set up his own service which would better reflect his ideas on care. He bought a large house – Normansfield – in south-west London, which he lived in with his family while developing residential accommodation in small rooms in the house and in extensions that were added over time. Support staff were attached to each small group, and were expected to live with them each day, sharing in meals and all activities, and sleeping in as required. Langdon Down and his family frequently ate meals and joined in activities with the people with learning difficulties. The idea was to replicate family care for those who could not live at home with other family members. Newspaper accounts published in the 1870s include the following:

> Normansfield is more like a home than a college or an institution. It has all the comforts and associations of a home. Good health of the patients remains the first consideration. Diet, regimen, cleanliness of person and clothing and the most skilful medical supervision are so minute and complete as seldom to fail. Training proceeds in an easy, natural and patient progress through helping and stimulating companionship, wholly free from the formality and rigour of the schools. The efficacy of the law of kindness has seldom been more strikingly illustrated. Discipline is maintained without

personal chastisement or material deprivation of any kind. No pupil is allowed to be shaken or slapped or deprived of food or subjected to any avengement. The duty laid on teachers and attendants is to gain the affection of their wards so fully that nothing will be to them a higher punishment than the disapprobation of their ministrants.

(Ward 1998)

Photographs of the 'patients' taken by Langdon Down show them to be immaculately dressed with smart hairstyles. Conor Ward in his biography (1998) says that 'residents of Normansfield were intended to live the lives of young ladies and gentlemen'. It is interesting to note the emphasis on good physical health; the White Paper (Department of Health 2001) also has a chapter (Chapter 6, p. 59) emphasising this. *Plus ça change . . .*!

At the beginning of the twentieth century the eugenics movement spread the idea that people with learning difficulties were a menace to the progress of society. Large numbers of people were locked up in large institutions, not for their benefit but to prevent them breeding and to keep them away from ordinary society. The notion of replicating family life was displaced by features of containment and ease of supervision, such as large dormitories. Overcrowding and lack of funding contributed to deterioration in the quality of care right up until scandals broke and were brought to public attention in the 1960s and 1970s. Initial responses to this situation were to 'tart up' the institutions with renovations, redecoration and recruitment of more staff. A programme of building smaller – but still large – 'hostels' was undertaken. It was not until the 1970s and beyond that the idea that had originally been proposed by Samuel Howe over a hundred years previously took root again: that people should live in very small numbers in ordinary houses.

Residential care as family-style home

Although Howe's ideas about the structure of residential services have found renewed allegiance today, Langdon Down's concept of residential care as replicating family life is not so clearly accepted. Confused views are prevalent about the purpose of residential care. Is it therapeutic, with planned training programmes to increase skills or reduce so-called 'challenging behaviour'? Is it primarily containment for people who cannot have an 'ordinary' home life? Or is it to support people in really having a true home and family base of their own?

Ironically, the idea of family life may be strongest in some of the remaining large congregations of people with learning difficulties in the form of self-contained communities (the White Paper calls them 'intentional communities'). It is possible for people there to have a strong sense of their home accommodation being a base for contribution to that community. In 1998, Angus Elliot, a man with learning difficulties who had lived at the Camphill Village Community at Botton, Yorkshire, for forty-two years, was awarded an MBE in the Queen's Birthday Honours List for services to that community. A vision for the future is that other people with learning difficulties will have opportunities to earn such a reward for service to an 'ordinary' community, through social inclusion rather than self-contained isolation. This latter feature of 'village communities' is illustrated by this extract from a poem by Tamar Segal describing Ravenswood Village in Berkshire:

> But to help you see us function
> We have a special way
> Of opening to the public:
> Our *annual* Open Day.
>> (quoted in Segal 1990, my emphasis; see also Lynn 2001)

Despite such isolation, the philosophy of family life and acceptance in such communities may have lessons for us. The L'Arche movement, founded by Jean Vanier, has a strong sense of its own 'community', sometimes well integrated into ordinary society and sometimes more self-contained (the communities in Britain are mostly in ordinary dispersed housing, but there is a larger 'village' at Trosly in France). Here are some expressions of the L'Arche philosophy, taken from the internet website of the American branch (http://www.larcheusa.org):

> We recognise the unique value of persons with a developmental disability to reveal that human suffering and joy can lead to growth, healing and unity. When their gift is received, individual, social and spiritual change occurs. We practise life sharing where persons with a mental disability and those who assist them live, work and pray together, creating a home. We develop relationships of mutuality in which people give and receive love. We create homes where faithful relationships based on forgiveness and celebration are nurtured. We seek to reveal the unique value and vocation of each person. We are active in changing society by choosing to live relationships in community as a sign of hope and love.

Family life provides a basis for self-esteem and confidence, for comfort and well-being and a sense of belonging, for practical support to do the things one wishes to do, for inclusion in the culture of one's inheritance and background and identity, and for acceptance and contribution and social inclusion in the local community.

Supporting residential care as family life

The primary intent of the principles of SRV is to maximise the chances of good relations between ordinary people and people at risk of social exclusion. Support workers in residential services are advocates for and companions of people with learning difficulties in this task. From the base of people's own homes, they are supported in presenting themselves to the local community in positive, contributing roles. These would include the roles of neighbour, family member, friend, customer of local services, home-dweller and citizen of the local community.

One of the lessons from application of PASSING, the service evaluation tool that is allied to SRV (Wolfensberger and Thomas 1983; Williams 1995b; see also Chapter 7), is that damage to the pursuit of positive social roles can easily be done quite unconsciously. Buildings, decor, furnishings, pictures, notices, etc. can all send out negative messages in their design, content or appearance – for example, that people are sick, or a nuisance, or childlike, or objects of fun and ridicule. Alternatively, by careful thought, such things can send out positive messages of contribution, responsibility, adulthood and good neighbourliness. A well-kept front garden can portray a positive message which can be ruined by careless upkeep, car parking, milkcrates, warning notices, nameplates identifying agency ownership, etc.

The closer the location is to ordinary community facilities for leisure, education, work, shopping, religious worship, pursuing hobbies and interests, etc., the greater will be the potential for social inclusion. As Langdon Down realised, if people with learning difficulties are to have the positive social reputation and status that should be theirs by right, they need strong support to present themselves well. A family-type home where there are loving relationships is the base for natural care and attention to cleanliness, dress, appearance and social graces.

The 'conservatism corollary' of SRV suggests that pursuing positive social roles requires much more than simply providing opportunities. Opening up equal opportunities is of course a necessary first step, but people with learning difficulties often have backgrounds of negative experiences and great disadvantages, as will be discussed later in this chapter. They are also at great risk of being thought of negatively by other people in society. The social model of disability (see Chapter 11) defines social inclusion, not just as physical presence in integrative social situations, but as being welcomed for the positive contribution that one makes to those situations. The concept of independence in this model is not of being able to do things unaided, but of having maximum support to do the things one wants to. Both SRV and the social model thus point to the need for strong support for people to achieve positive social roles and genuine inclusion in social activities for the contribution that people bring. Support workers need to have a powerful sense of the positive characteristics and beneficial social contribution of each person they support, and to see their task as providing maximum support to the person in presenting those characteristics and making that contribution in social settings.

For most people, home is not a place where they shut themselves in isolation and seclusion. In any event, it is not in the best interests of people at risk of social exclusion to adopt this concept of home. Rather, home can be the base for social intercourse – for example for entertaining friends and for providing hospitality to relatives. These things will not happen unless support staff facilitate them. An adult in their own home should be able to invite friends and relatives to visit, offer them meals and refreshments, share activities with them there, and ideally have accommodation available where they can stay.

In ways like these we can map out what true family home life might be like for adults with learning difficulties. Most importantly, it will be highly individualised depending on the cultural identity and the interests of the person, and this requires flexibility (Thomas 1999). Aspects of the structure and management of residential services can, however, easily stand in the way of successful pursuit of this. Hierarchical structures of management, excessive rules and regulations, an attitude of complete risk-avoidance, and a crippling burden of record-keeping and form-filling, are common factors that sap the energy and destroy creativity. Supportive management structures will seek ways of minimising these pressures. For example, Hall *et al.* (1996) describe a non-hierarchical system of teamwork in which all support team members play equal roles for equal pay with equal responsibilities; this gets away completely from the common notion that there must be a 'person-in-charge', even in the context of supporting someone in their own home! At wider organisational level, good management should be seen as facilitation of creativity and commitment and a sense of responsible freedom by employees, not as tight control of every activity through excessive record-keeping and monitoring. Disasters are best prevented through close, caring relationships that naturally protect vulnerable people from harm; there is much evidence that they are not prevented by bureaucratic procedures.

The need for family-style care

In this chapter a picture is being painted of support relationships for small groups of people in ordinary houses that give them a sense of having their own family life in a place that is their own home. Support that tries to achieve this should derive from an understanding of the needs of each person, and a strong sense of why this family-type relationship and support is necessary for them.

People with learning difficulties are often defined in terms of their behaviour. Many means have been devised to assess the 'skill deficits' or 'challenging behaviour' of people. Such assessments often define the lifestyles and opportunities available to people. Sometimes they lead to oppressive 'programmes' of planned activities and teaching imposed on people in their own homes. Ironically, it is possible that the concentration of research and development resources in recent years on the perceived problem of 'challenging behaviour' has led to the cat-egorisation of much larger numbers of those receiving support as 'people with challenging behaviour' than would otherwise have been the case. The more investment in treatment, the more prevalent the problem!

Supporters of a family-type home life for people with learning difficulties serve those people better if they focus not on behaviour but on experiences. Some frameworks for doing this have been helpfully developed in recent years, for example 'Person-Centred Planning' (O'Brien and O'Brien 1998; Sanderson *et al.* 1998). The White Paper *Valuing People* (Department of Health 2001) proposes the widespread introduction of Person-Centred Planning as a means of involving people in the assessment of their needs. The best provider services already use this or equivalent methods, but it is difficult to see how it can be implemented in the context of care management (at present many people with severe learning difficulties, especially those in long-term care, do not have a care manager at all, let alone a sophisticated care management assessment method).

In Person-Centred Planning, information sought about individuals who are supported, in order to understand their needs, includes:

What is the person's story?
What and who are important to the person?
What is life like now?
What are the person's gifts?
What are their dreams and nightmares?
What is the person's reputation?
What is their identity?

A similar approach is based on a more thorough appreciation of a person's life experiences. These can be reviewed in a number of areas of life: family relationships, community relationships, economic status, experience of choice, experience of key life stages such as birth or starting school or leaving home, effects of impairment, and future to look forward to (Williams 1995b). Many people will have experienced fraught family relationships and enforced separation from family, although their family may remain of great importance to them. Many people will have had negative experience of community relationships, including rejection by individuals and by social agencies such as schools or leisure facilities; some people may have had little contact with ordinary community members or facilities. Many people are likely to have always been materially poor, with few resources within their ownership or control. Many people may never have experienced choice, even in simple areas like dress or food. For many people, experiences of key life events will have been negative: their birth may well have been seen as a disaster rather than a cause for celebration; starting school may have meant exclusion from the neighbourhood school and separation from friends and brothers and sisters; leaving home may have been an enforced and traumatic event leading to loss of contact with family. The consequences of impairment might mean difficulty in communicating needs, non-achievement of things one would like to have achieved, or dependence on others who are often unreliable. The only future to look forward to may always have been bleak: continuing isolation, discomfort and vulnerability to hurt and oppression.

Support workers have an opportunity, through relationship-building in the context of family-like home life, to compensate for such negative experiences as these. In addition, people may need long-term and patient condolence and support with deep emotional upset at their internalised perception of themselves as 'impaired' and 'a problem' (see Sinason 1992). This concept – that people with learning difficulties may be 'wounded' in spirit as a result of internalisation of negative relationships towards them and perceptions of them by others – is central to Jean Vanier's 'life-sharing' model of care expressed in the philosophy of L'Arche (Clarke 1974; see also Williams 2001 and Chapter 12). It is also reflected in this passage by Bengt Nirje, one of the founders of the concept of 'normalisation':

> The awareness of being handicapped, the insight into being mentally retarded, is expressed in possibly distorted self-concepts or defeated utterances or through defence mechanisms, closing in on inner sorrows. To assert yourself, in your own eyes or before your family, and to confront society – friends, neighbours, co-workers or people in general – might be difficult for anyone, but the awareness of being handicapped brings a complicating factor – the problem of understanding oneself. And in the end, even the retarded person has to manage as a private person and has to define himself before others in the circumstances of his life and existence.
>
> (Nirje 1980)

So the task of residential care is to provide a home and family-type care and support to enable people to have good experiences that compensate for past disadvantage and oppression, to have positive social roles that bring about genuine social inclusion based on welcoming identity and contribution, and to comfort and empathise with the emotional 'wounds' of the internalisation of negative perceptions.

Supporting supporters

This specification is no mean task! To pursue it we must recruit people prepared to make commitments to individual people and to be comfortable with long-term, often unclear, objectives. The requirement is for warmth and identification with people's humanity. Training for support workers should include a major element on values, identification and equality, and a social family-like approach to people's needs. Unfortunately, resources for such training are easily usurped by ever-growing statutory requirements, often deriving from European legislation. The majority of training nowadays is in areas such as health and safety, manual handling, food hygiene, risk assessment, and control and restraint. While of course these topics are important, there needs to be a strong underlying base of values and positive relationships that will naturally protect people from harm.

Training in values, and having values as the basis of supervision and management of support workers, also help to focus team members on the rights and needs of those they support and care for, rather than excessively on their own rights in employment. The best teams function with a sense that it is a privilege to work with people with learning difficulties, that it is enjoyable, and that the relationships involved can be integrated into one's life as a whole. Within a context of concern by organisations for the welfare and comfort of their employees, which is of course good and necessary, this attitude will foster flexibility, commitment and devotion, and will reduce excessive concern with monetary rewards, time off and exceptional conditions of work. Family-style home support can only be provided in this way.

Two stories of 'challenging behaviour'

This story comes from my own experience. Elizabeth came to live in a house where she was cared for by a team of support workers. Previously she had spent time in a 'behavioural unit', following which she had refused any possessions. She would not have curtains at her window, her room was completely bare, and she even destroyed her clothes if they were kept in her room. She was very reluctant to leave the house and when she did she often had outbursts of temper in public places. The support team suspected that this behaviour was partly a reaction to the taking away of control over her possessions and activities in the 'behavioural' programme, and partly an expression of anger arising from her realisation that she had impairments and was thought of negatively by other people. They embarked on a long-term task of offering and respecting choice, gradually introducing her to new experiences at her own pace of acceptance, showing consistent positive regard for her in all circumstances, and treating her as an adult with family-style relationships and activities in her own home. Gradually over a number of years Elizabeth became more tolerant of furnishings, curtains, pictures on the wall and homely decor. She became more enthusiastic about going out, especially to places or activities she chose herself. She was helped to build up and retain friendships and acquaintances with a wide range of people who liked her. Contact with her parents was maintained and strengthened, partly by the offering of hospitality to them by Elizabeth in her home, and by the provision of transport to get there, as might be provided by any adult son or daughter. It took years to re-establish Elizabeth's trust in other people and her ability to enjoy herself without 'testing' the strength of people's relationships with her. The transformation in her after these years, however, has been great, and it is likely to be more permanent than the effects of any short-term 'behavioural' programme.

The second story comes from the account of L'Arche by Clarke (1974):

> The role of the assistants is one of a peaceful and non-violent presence to absorb some of the anguish of the handicapped that a life of rejection has engendered in them. I began to realise that any resistance to David was a kind of violence that only added another link to the whole chain of violence in which he was a victim. So I adopted an attitude of greater receptivity and non-violence towards him, allowing him to do as he pleased with me. The first thing that I discovered once I stopped resisting him was that a great deal of tension went out of me. I could now adopt a very simple and consistent openness to him. I found myself no longer avoiding his company. But rather seeking him out just for the pleasure of being with him. Although nothing seemed to have changed in his attitude towards me, something had changed quite considerably in me by virtue of the gift I had received to no longer resist

his aggressive activity. Now it mattered much less to me that David change. I wanted him to grow, but my love for him was not on the condition that he grow and be different than he was. I could accept him much more just as he was. In the lowering of some of my own barriers of aggression and self-preservation, the two of us came much closer together. With this greater closeness I could see much more of the goodness and beauty of his person, which one could scarcely fail to love.

These stories illustrate the long-term nature of residential support, and the acceptance of people that is required for true family-like home life.

Serendipity

Serendip is an old name for Sri Lanka. There is a story of three princes who set out to find a treasure there. They never found it, but on the way they found many unexpected things that gave them equal pleasure. The accidental discovery of good things has come to be called 'serendipity'.

There is a current tendency towards trying to define all work with people with learning difficulties in terms of specific predictable objectives, preferably measurable with a stated time for achievement (so-called SMART goals – specific, measurable, achievable, resourced and time-bound). However, the stories above illustrate that the outcomes of support for people cannot always be predicted. Services need to accept that often goals will be uncertain and may never be achieved. Processes of care and support that are based on relationships and values, and that seek to compensate for negative past experiences, have a value in their own right.

If we can get away from notions of specific objectives, and aim for a more nebulous family-style home life, then there will be frequent instances of serendipity. People will show unexpected progress; they will show unforeseen strengths, perhaps particularly in areas of concern for others; they will form strong relationships with unpredictable mutual benefits; their humanity will show through at unexpected times of difficulty.

The following story is again from my own experience. Stan lives in a small house with the help of a support team. He has had some hard experiences of separation from his family and unsupportive actions by them, and he also has a recognition of his impairment and the fact that others think negatively of him. As a result he is very emotionally insecure and, like Elizabeth described above, destroys his possessions as an expression of distress. A few years ago, it was suggested that he might take part in a teaching session about people with learning difficulties on a course for nurses at a nearby university. Stan showed enthusiasm for this, and the visit was arranged. He was accompanied by a support worker from his home. The expectation was that Stan would remain meek and uncommunicative, but that the students would benefit from meeting him and that Stan would enjoy meeting them. In the event, Stan asked many questions of the students about their life, and was taken on a tour of the campus by the students. He spoke freely and articulately about himself, and with affection about the friends he lives with. He had moved easily into the role of 'visiting lecturer' and his achievement there was a source of pride to himself and his supporter. He is now regularly invited to contribute to the training course.

Mission and vision in residential services

As well as living easily with the concept of serendipity, organisations and individuals providing residential services and support should have consistent and coherent ideas of their mission, and a vision of the future they are aiming for. Most services express allegiance to what have become known as the 'five accomplishments' delineated by John O'Brien (1987): community presence, choice, respect, competence and community participation (see Chapter 12). John O'Brien, however, did not intend these concepts to be a blueprint for services to slavishly follow. He devised a process called 'Framework for Accomplishment' which enables people to learn about the life experiences, wishes and needs of individuals and then devise parameters for service design that set appropriate 'accomplishments' depending on the understanding gained about those specific individuals. Few services that subscribe to the 'five accomplishments' have been through this process that tells them *why* such accomplishments are important for the specific people they support. The basis of most statements of allegiance to the 'five accomplishments' is thus extremely weak.

Services must go through a process of understanding the experiences, needs and wishes of the unique individual people they support. People hanker after 'blueprints' for the development of services, but it is crucial that both purchasing and providing agencies carry out sensitive and individualised processes of discovering the specific needs of individuals. In mission statements, these processes should be as prominent as the outcomes that are striven for, and the vision should be that the processes will operate so that each person has experiences that compensate for past disadvantage, increase self-esteem, ease hurt and anger, engender trust in others and enable people to express their gifts and contribution to society.

Rather than simply stating the 'five accomplishments' in a mission statement, a residential service should include statements of process. Examples might include:

- that there will be a holistic assessment of needs;
- that the positive identity and skills and characteristics and achievements of the people supported will be celebrated;
- that people will be supported to plan for and take control of their lives to the greatest extent possible;
- that there will be understanding of the life experiences of the people supported that constitute oppression or disablement, and that the service will counteract these experiences and compensate for them; and

- that good family-like relationships of caring and equality and adulthood will be modelled and promoted.

Some helpful frameworks have been devised for developing a vision of the future for individual people, for example PATH (Planning Alternative Tomorrows with Hope – Pearpoint *et al.* 1992). The White Paper *Valuing People* (Department of Health 2001) is worded in a way that supports these processes in principle, but the depth of understanding of the implications might be questioned (the bibliography in the White Paper, for example, is disappointingly narrow and limited). The good principles can so easily be lost through insufficient resources and over-bureaucratisation of services.

Day services

So far in this chapter I have said little about day services. In the introductory summary the continuing rather chaotic state of day services was touched on. There remains confusion about the aims of services and appropriate service structures and designs that can meet those aims. An analysis of current issues in day services for people with learning difficulties is given by Williams (1995a). As mentioned earlier, the White Paper (Department of Health 2001) proposes a five-year modernisation of day services, but contains no real analysis of the fundamental problems they face.

Daytime services should work in close collaboration with families and home support services. Although this would be unusual for ordinary adults, people with learning difficulties are vulnerable to lack of consistency and differences in values between services they receive. All services for individual people with learning difficulties should respect each other's role and work in close co-operation with each other. Thus, all the considerations about residential work in this chapter should be appreciated and subscribed to by day services.

Day services, however, can validly have much more specific functions and can adopt support methods and practices that would be inappropriate in the family-style home life that I have described. If in future there is proper separation of work preparation and support services, education services, leisure and social support services, and therapeutic or treatment services, each of these will be able to develop efficient methods. Appropriate personnel can be appointed, with specific training and qualifications, to provide specific support in appropriate places with appropriate tools. If all services are pursuing social inclusion, it can be expected that most services will provide support in integrative situations rather than in special settings.

Which services are required by an individual person will depend on an individualised process of determining need. Guidelines for this process, together with a wide range of examples of innovative and creative development of daytime opportunities are given by McIntosh and Whittaker (1998). The White Paper's commitment to Person-Centred Planning will also help if it can be implemented.

When people have interesting and contributive daytime activities as well as a high-quality family-style home life, then they have a strong personal base for pursuit of their right to be seen and treated in society as equal and valued citizens.

References

Carter, J. (1981) *Day Services for Adults: Somewhere to Go*, London, Allen and Unwin.

Clarke, B. (1974) *Enough Room for Joy: Jean Vanier's L'Arche – A Message for Our Time*, London, Darton, Longman and Todd.

Dagnan, D. and Drewett, R. (1988) Community based care for people with a mental handicap: a family placement scheme in County Durham, *British Journal of Social Work*, 18: 543–575.

Department of Health (1999) *Facing the Facts: Services for People with Learning Disabilities – A Policy Impact Study of Social Care and Health Services*, London, The Stationery Office.

Department of Health (2001) *Valuing People: A New Strategy for Learning Disability for the 21st Century*, London, The Stationery Office.

Emerson, E., Robertson, J., Hatton, C., Gregory, N., Kessissoglou, S., Hallam, A., Knapp, M., Jarbrink, K., Netten, A., Walsh, P.N., Linehan, C., Hillery, J. and Durkan, J. (1999) *Quality and Costs of Residential Supports for People with Learning Disabilities: Summary Report*, Manchester, Hester Adrian Research Centre, University of Manchester.

Ferrity, B., Ford, D. and Bratt, A. (1986) The private sector: just landladies or carers? *Mental Handicap*, 14: 166–169.

Flynn, M. (1989) *Independent Living for Adults with Mental Handicap: A Place of My Own*, London, Cassell.

Hall, B., Jones, T. and Williams, P. (1996) Collective team management in a community support service, *Elders – the Journal of Care and Practice*, 5(2), 41–51.

Heron, A. (1982) *Better Services for the Mentally Handicapped? Lessons from the Sheffield Evaluation Studies*, London, King's Fund Centre.

Holman, A. and Bewley, C. (1999) *Funding Freedom 2000: People with Learning Difficulties using Direct Payments*, London, Values Into Action.

Lynn, S. (2001) Ravenswood: village ghetto or thriving community?, *Community Living*, 14(4): 14–16.

McIntosh, B. and Whittaker, A. (1998) *Days of Change: a Practical Guide to Developing Better Day Opportunities with People with Learning Difficulties*, London, King's Fund Publishing.

Nirje, B. (1980) The normalisation principle. In: R. Flynn and K. Nitsch (eds) *Normalisation, Social Integration and Community Services*, Baltimore, University Park Press.

O'Brien, J. (1987) A guide to lifestyle planning. In: B. Wilcox and T. Bellamy (eds) *A Comprehensive Guide to the Activities Catalogue*, Baltimore, Paul Brookes.

O'Brien, J. and O'Brien, C.L. (eds) (1998) *A Little Book about Person Centred Planning*, Toronto, Inclusion Press.

Pearpoint, J., O'Brien, J. and Forest, M. (1992) *PATH – Planning Alternative Tomorrows with Hope*, Toronto, Inclusion Press.

Race, D. (1999) *Social Role Valorization and the English Experience*, London, Whiting and Birch.

Sanderson, H., Kennedy, J., Ritchie, P. and Goodwin, G. (1998) *People, Plans and Possibilities*, Edinburgh, SHS Ltd.

Segal, S.S. (ed.) (1990) *The Place of Special Villages and Residential Communities*, Bicester, A B Academic Publishers.

Sinason, V. (1992) *Mental Handicap and the Human Condition*, London, Free Association Books.

Thomas, R.R. (1999) *Building a House for Diversity: How a Fable about a Giraffe and an Elephant Offers New Strategies for Today's Workforce*, New York, American Management Association.

Ward, O.C. (1998) *John Langdon Down: A Caring Pioneer*, London, Royal Society of Medicine Press.

Williams, P. (1995a) Residential and day services. In: N. Malin (ed.) *Services for People with Learning Disabilities*, London, Routledge.

Williams, P. (1995b) The PASS and PASSING evaluation instruments. In: D. Pilling and G. Watson (eds) *Evaluating Quality in Services for Disabled and Older People*, London, Jessica Kingsley.

Williams, P. (1995c) The results from PASS and PASSING evaluations. In: D. Pilling and G. Watson (eds) *Evaluating Quality in Services for Disabled and Older People*, London, Jessica Kingsley.

Williams, P. (2001) Social role valorisation and the concept of 'wounds', *Clinical Psychology Forum*, 149: 6–8.

Wolfensberger, W. (1975) *The Origin and Nature of Our Institutional Models*, Syracuse, New York, Human Policy Press.

Wolfensberger, W. (1998) *A Brief Introduction to Social Role Valorisation*, third edition, Syracuse, New York, Training Institute, Syracuse University.

Wolfensberger, W. and Thomas, S. (1983) *PASSING – Programme Analysis of Service Systems' Implementation of Normalization Goals*, 2nd edition, Toronto, NIMR.

Chapter 4

Education Services

Why segregated special schools must close

Joe Whittaker and John Kenworthy

Introduction

To exclude people described as having learning difficulties from mainstream local schools, colleges and universities is an injustice. (NB: We use the term 'described as having learning difficulties'. We do not accept the term 'people *with* learning difficulties', as these 'difficulties' are socially constructed. Assessments and labels used to define individuals are oppressive. Therefore we use the term to describe people's experience in the present schooling system. We look forward to a time when we can write about 'learners' who are valued equally.) Such an injustice demands that we look more creatively at the way we operate within existing educational systems, that we challenge the regulations that control admissions procedures for people described as having learning difficulties and we revolutionise our understanding of 'special education'. We have to find different ways of hearing what learners want to learn and different ways of learning together. We have to acknowledge that the present system of selecting some individuals *out* of education is at best an ineffective use of our resources and at worst an abuse of individual learners. We cannot wait for an attitude change or general consensus before we enforce the right, by legislation, of all learners to belong and participate in mainstream educational provision. Segregated education and the resulting denial of human rights can no longer be an option if we are to have an inclusive education agenda.

We will examine how the history of segregation, the practice of labelling and the denial of rights of learners have together stifled a dynamic shift towards inclusive education. We will also consider the powerful factors which maintain the segregated school and some of the common doubts and fears about an inclusive system. Finally, we look towards the future possibility of a fair and just education system in which the rights of all learners are safeguarded. Implicit in this is the view that an inclusive system cannot, by definition, co-exist with segregated schools and that the closure of special schools and the redistribution of their massive resources is the necessary precondition for the inclusion of all learners. We place these arguments in the context of Human Rights legislation (Human Rights Act 1998), the White Paper *Valuing People* (DoH 2001) and other government initiatives which appear to promote an inclusive agenda.

Compulsory segregation

Since the 1950s successive Education Acts and government advice have promoted the 'integration' of people described as having learning difficulties. (Anderson 1973). Indeed, the Warnock Report (DES 1978), which underpinned the 1981 Education Act, was hailed as the 'integrationist charter' at the time of its publication. However, the percentage of the total school population in segregated special schools in England has not changed dramatically since 1980. In 1981, 127,157 children were in segregated special schools (DfEE 2000). In 2000, 94,142 children were in segregated special schools and 8,479 children were placed in 'referral units'. This is surprising, as the promise of the 1981 Education Act and successive legislation was that over a period of years there would be more integration of children into mainstream schools *not* that more children would be processed as having special educational needs. Considering the rhetoric of support for social inclusion in general and inclusive education in particular, from the present government (DfE 1997), these figures should be a cause for concern. It is certainly alarming there are still 102,621 pupils in segregated schooling, suggesting that segregation remains the touchstone of 'special education'.

While we appear to have legislation promoting inclusive education for people described as having learning difficulties, it does not mean that their inclusion is guaranteed. There exists within our educational system powerful forces, which will work to prevent such reforms.

The 1981 Education Act not only promoted greater integration but introduced the 'Statement of Special Educational Needs' (SEN). This placed a formal obligation on local education authorities (LEAs) to provide a written account of the child's identified need, the provision they would make to meet that need and the school placement they would offer. At the time of its introduction the Statement appeared to offer children and parents real consultation, greater access to main-stream education and more creative and comprehensive support. However, for many families 'statementing' has proved to be a painful and laborious process in which their child is categorised and labelled. Local Authorities then use the Statement to legitimise the rejection and exclusion of the child from their local neighbourhood schools. Thus, for these families the Statement has not opened doors to new opportunities for their children but rather has served notice that the mainstream school doors remain firmly closed.

According to government statistics (DfEE 2000) 3 per cent of the school population in England now have Statements of SEN. The number of Statements continues to rise. In the year 2000 the number rose from 248,041 pupils to 252,857. Forty per cent of these children with Statements continue to be segregated in special schools or units. This process continues to direct large numbers of children into special schools and units because segregation remains the powerful orthodoxy, which has a critical influence on the outcome of the assessment process.

It can be demonstrated that even when children with a particular label are successfully supported in mainstream schools, the statementing process can reconstruct other categories and attach new labels to a new group of learners (Tomlinson 1982; Wade and Moore 1993). The labels can have spurious suffixes like 'spectrum', 'syndrome' or 'challenging'. Such terms give the eventual label added gravitas and serve to justify a segregated special school place. Segregated special schools develop like an amoeba, reforming to accommodate the 'reconstructed special pupil'. Special schools continue to use names which reflect the natural beauty of the countryside. 'The Elms', 'Woodside', 'Beech Tree House', 'Moorbrook', 'The Oaks', typify the leafy names which serve as camouflage for their purpose, which is to separate large numbers of children from their own natural communities and schools.

The statementing process is incorporated within the 'Code of Practice' (DfE 1994b). The procedures are designed to assess and identify a child's particular support requirements in five stages.

Stages 1–3 are school based, with support coming from specialists outside the school at stage 3. Stage 4 involves the LEA giving consideration to a formal assessment of a child's SEN and Stage 5 is the preparation of a formal statement from a multi-disciplinary team. The detail of the Code of Practice and the statementing process is also under consideration by government as this is written. However, it remains uncertain whether the revised procedures will promote appropriate support for the individual child to attend their local mainstream school or whether they will continue to be used by LEAs and head teachers to restrict access to these schools.

The Statement of SEN and the Code of Practice continues to put the learner under the 'spotlight' and gives professional assessments a disproportionate influence in relation to the parent's or the child's views. Assessment procedures too often define the child's need by attempting to 'scientifically' quantify or categorise 'the child's difficulty or problem'. These 'difficulties' might be psychological, medical, cognitive or behavioural characteristics. Once the measurements have been 'objectively' gathered, they are discussed at multi-disciplinary meetings by a gathering of professionals, some of whom may have never met the child in question. These professional assessments continue to focus on the individual learner's 'failings' rather than on the shortcomings of the educational support systems available. The assessments are invariably norm-based, where inappropriate and meaningless comparisons are made with other children of the same chronological, developmental or even 'mental' age. It is here that the child's difference is constructed and the path to segregation and rejection justified.

Segregation is the most likely outcome of statementing when the following conditions apply:

Where the LEA making the Statement is committed to maintaining a segregated special school sector

There is a wide and well-documented variation between LEAs with comparable demographics and total school populations in terms of both the percentage of pupils they statement and the percentage of special school places they provide. LEAs which maintain a relatively high percentage of statements do not necessarily provide a relatively high percentage of segregated special school places and vice versa. The evidence, which is freely available from LEAs in their annual 'Section 42 Statements', suggests that the number of segregated special school places provided by an LEA is fairly arbitrary and determined largely by local historical and political factors. For the child who is being statemented this means that, in some instances, they may be up to two to three times more likely to be segregated in a special school in one LEA than they would if they lived in a neighbouring authority (Kenworthy 1997).

That the descriptions of the child's needs in Section 2 of the Statement rely heavily on norm-based assessment procedures

The advantage of developmental, intelligence and literacy tests is that they provide the time-pressed professional with a clear and concise procedure which allows certain 'expert' (i.e. difficult to challenge) judgements to be made. However, the weakness of norm-based assessment is that the child's needs and idiosyncrasies remain poorly defined. Instead a measure of their abilities relative to their age–peer group is used to point out how unacceptably different the child is. Thus, assessment reports and statements which rely heavily on norm-based assessment tend to stress the child's negative difference from the 'average child'. This language of difference does not accurately describe individuals' ability and needs but rather focuses on inability, deficiency and dysfunction. When the degree of negative difference needs to be emphasised the lexicon of difference is found to include 'severe', 'profound', 'complex', 'multiple', etc.

That the provision identified to meet the child's needs in Part 3 of the Statement tends to emphasise resources and arrangements, which are not typically available in the LEA mainstream schools

Assessments based on performance criteria tend to pose questions such as 'What are his/her abilities/strengths in these areas?' and 'What specific sort of provision does she/he need to help her/him to advance in this area?' While many professionals, particularly teachers, routinely use performance-based assessment, it is the insidious culture of norm-based assessment in statementing which allows provision to be described in broad and essentially meaningless phrases. We have many examples of statements which include phrases such as: 'a quiet, distraction free environment'; 'to receive teaching in small groups'; 'access to a broad, balanced and relevant curriculum suitably modified to meet his/her needs' and 'support from staff experienced in working with children with severe learning difficulties'. It is not difficult to see how each of the learners who were the subjects of these Statements came to be directed to segregated schools.

The present education law (DfE 1994) says that a child has special educational needs if they require special help. The law states that if a child finds it much harder to learn than other children of the same age or if they have a disability which means they cannot use the normal educational facilities, then 'special provision' is required. The present law discriminates by presenting the individual child as the 'problem', whereas a legal obligation ought to be placed on the LEA and school to provide the appropriate supports to enable the child to participate and learn with their group of peers. Destructive, unreliable and meaningless comparisons with other learners based on the mythical 'normal' or 'average' child do not have any validity in a genuinely inclusive process of assessment and education.

Learners without labels – historical issues

It is often argued that we need labels and statements to direct the appropriate resources and support to the particular learner. This is indeed part of the distortion and legacy of a system which is based upon the false premise that it is the 'individual's difficulty', rather than the system's deficiencies, which prevents full and active participation of individuals. However, it is important to acknowledge that the present ritual of statementing a child or the attachment of a particular label to that child, is no guarantee that the appropriate support and resources will be provided for the child. Appropriate support should not be seen as an 'optional extra' or dependent on 'good will' or for 'expert delivery only'. Supports should be so effective and available that they are not recognised or presented as 'special'. A ventilator, a signer, an interpreter, a personal assistant, voice recognition software, physical adaptations, accessible transport and toilet facilities should be as available and as central to meaningful learning environments as a pair of spectacles or a teacher.

The preoccupation with assessing the individual learner and in particular those described as having learning difficulties is an educational cul-de-sac. Such an approach has evolved from a medical model of testing–diagnosis–treatment. The same medical approach has been adopted and applied to the development of some individuals' learning experiences, as discussed in Chapter 2. Mind, intelligence and capacity for learning are often presented as the same 'entity' and are presented in the form of numerical scores and attached to individuals. Such scores have been used, or more accurately, misused, within our schooling system throughout the past century to divide people, by valuing some and devaluing others. A classic reference in medical literature reflects some of the mythology about people who experience 'learning difficulties' (Tredgold 1963). The text provides a useful insight into the use of tests and the applications used to measure individuals. Such measurements continue to be used to give legitimacy to the segregation and rejection of individuals. Tredgold (1963: 2) suggests tests are applied in such a way that 'their results can be expressed in numbers – which is comforting and appears respectably scientific, or scientifically respectable'. Such numerical assessments have led to a clear self-fulfilling prophecy. From the same book one can read the pattern of assumptions being constructed in the observations made by professionals on individuals who had been 'tested' and labelled as 'defectives':

> Three nice-looking defective children, sisters and brothers, who at times appear models of propriety, they had all the characteristics of little demons. With innocent expressions they would furtively accomplish the most abominable mischief, and after meekly acknowledging the error of their ways, would emphasise their apology by a missile flung at the head of the person who had attempted to bring them repentance. When they grow up, children like these may commit serious crimes such as incendiarism, train wrecking, criminal assaults upon little girls and homicide. Although these acts at times appear to be sudden and unpremeditated, they may show evidence of previous deliberation and plan, and sometimes of cunning to avoid detection, though at a low level.
>
> (Tredgold 1963: 255)

Throughout the history of medicine such an evident fear of difference has allowed dangerous assumptions to be made by professionals about the essential humanity of their 'subjects'. When the status and power of professionals is underpinned by a notion that they are in possession of a higher 'mind' or morality, higher 'intelligence' and greater 'capacity for learning', it has been possible for horrific and dehumanising procedures to be inflicted on disabled people in the guise of scientific respectability (*Science and the Swastika*, Channel 4, 2001). From experiments in the death camps to 'subnormality hospitals' and 'ESN' schools, medicine has a great deal to answer for, not the least of which is the legacy of segregation that is still embraced by our education systems.

Professionals can disempower and devalue people who experience learning in ways that they don't appreciate or may not understand. Categorising and labelling individuals in the process of their learning is also a very powerful way of controlling an individual's opportunity for learning. To quantify such a 'learning experience' with numerical tests and a variety of pseudo-scientific labels tells us nothing of value or can never give meaning to an individual learner's experience. The only meaningful label to describe the individual in a learning environment is that person's name (Biklen 1992). It is only when we are able to make connections with Azis, Alison or Navin rather than 'the autistic child', 'the one on Ritalin', 'the EBD child' or the 'bright one' that we can begin to create and understand a learning environment that is meaningful and productive for all learners.

Personal accounts taken from individuals who have experienced segregated education (Rae 1999) highlight the damage done to individuals, families and communities when we segregate some children from their peers. We have come to know that segregation in childhood leads to segregation in further education, housing, employment and adult relationships. Martin Luther King was quoted as saying 'segregation was the illicit offspring of an intercourse between injustice and immorality'.

Again, Chapter 2 notes how compulsory incarceration in long-stay 'mental subnormality' institutions many miles away from their families and communities was a defining feature of services to people described as having learning difficulties during the twentieth century. In many long-stay institutions, even in the 1970s, it was not uncommon for very young children to live in wards alongside wards for adult and elderly disabled people (Thomas and Ryan 1987). Another common feature of these 'mental subnormality hospitals' was the hospital school which children from the wards together with children from the surrounding area would attend. A common view at the time was that some children needed institutional care and/or education in a hospital school because they 'would never cope' in a family or in an 'ordinary' special school. Thankfully following the reforms of the 1970s and 1980s, children described as having learning difficulties are no longer placed in dilapidated Victorian institutions or expected to attend hospital schools. However, the thinking which underpinned the existence of these places still has a powerful influence on contemporary thinking. It is crucial to recognise the link between the medical model of social care of the past century and the medical/ therapeutic model of education which the segregated special schooling system still enshrines. The continued use of diagnostic labels is one of the clearest ways in which this is manifested.

It would appear that the one constant in the permutation of variables in the field of learning disabilities is the number of segregated places available. If we retain 100,000 places we will process 100,000 learners with appropriate labels, appropriate justifications, supported by appropriate professional rationale to fill the places available. The processes we adopt will not be guided by a child's particular support requirements to join their local communities. Rather, they will be driven by the need to feed the machine which is the segregated special school system.

Rights of appeal

Education law as it currently stands still results in compulsory segregation of large numbers of children described as having learning difficulties. The existing legislation gives LEAs the power to send a child to a segregated special school against the child's and the parent's wishes if they, the LEA, judge it to be the appropriate way of meeting the child's 'special' needs. The LEA is legally obliged to take this course if they conclude that the placement of a child in their local mainstream school would be:

- inconsistent with meeting the child's needs;
- adversely affecting the learning of 'others'; or
- an inefficient use of resources.

These three caveats are due for change in a new SEN and Disability Bill, which received Royal assent before the 2001 general election. The intention is to 'strengthen' the rights of parents to choose mainstream school by removing two of the above conditions. However, it is intended to retain the second condition, which will oblige the LEA to forcibly segregate a child who experiences learning difficulties if they are said to adversely affect the learning of other children. This sort of conditional inclusion is unacceptable and will continue to be used by those with a vested interest in retaining segregated provision to reject and isolate children described as having learning difficulties.

Parents will continue to have a right of appeal, when they disagree with the LEA, including an application to a so-called independent special educational needs tribunal. However, rejection is too often the experience for many parents who have sat before this tribunal and asked for a mainstream place for their child. The notion of the SEN tribunal being 'independent' should be fundamentally challenged. The composition of the 'independent' SEN tribunal when introduced, in 1996, was overwhelmingly comprised of non-disabled professionals for whom the 'segregated special school' remained a powerful, if not the only, orthodoxy (Whittaker and Crabtree 1997). This can be verified through examination of the decisions of tribunals (Jordans 2000) and the callous dismissal of the arguments for mainstream education for individual families by the law courts. The Cranes and McKibben families who have struggled to have their children included within their local mainstream schools over many years of bitter struggle provide painful testimony and clear justification for an end to the existing ritual of appeal (Brandon 1997; Kenworthy and Whittaker 2000). It is also an anachronism that this, so-called independent, 'quango' is given the power to accept or reject the right of a child to attend their local mainstream school. Such a situation is comparable to a professional body, consisting of white Afrikaans in South Africa, deciding the schooling of a black child in a schooling system established and maintained for white learners, prior to the obscenity of apartheid being overthrown.

Any education legislation which intends to move beyond the rhetoric of inclusive education has to remove all the conditions of entry to the mainstream provision for pupils described as having learning difficulties, while simultaneously bringing about the systematic ending of all segregated provision. The discrimination of people described as having learning difficulties is not an educational issue. It is much more an issue of the human right of the child to make a responsible contri-bution to their school and community (Barnes 1991; Campbell and Oliver 1996). The history, values and continued promotion of segregated services in the field of learning disabilities is a clear testimony to a corrupt provision in general, and a lack of wisdom in our education system in particular.

Equality, rights and advocacy

The change required within the educational system cannot be seen in isolation either from the wider political context or from the human rights debate. Effective inclusion of learners cannot and should not be a choice. It is necessary to right an injustice. It is urgent that we work more creatively to end such injustices. The UN's Salamanca Statement (Salamanca 1994) provided a valuable action plan for the rights of the child and was a positive contribution to a more inclusive agenda where ninety countries with 400 delegates signed up to comprehensive human rights in education across the world.

Those who have traditionally been excluded from mainstream education are beginning to give leadership in the struggle for inclusive education (Rae 1999; Finklestein 2000). Such a powerful struggle to end the injustice of segregated education can be related to historical struggles of other disenfranchised groups (Bunch and Valeo 1998). One aspect of the women's struggle to bring about equality was to end their exclusion from university education. It was almost eighty years of struggle before women gained access to university. Initially women were denied access because it was 'scientifically proven' that their brains were 'too small'. It was argued that women could not manage such a high level of studying, they would not be able to operate within the enormity of university life and it would create hysteria for women, affecting their reproductive systems and consequently affect their ability to produce children. This would have a damaging effect upon the population. After a bitter struggle women eventually did start to undertake university study in the 1870s. However, in the early stages they had to have a chaperone when attending lectures and had to wait in an ante-room near the lecture theatre until the lecture proper started. For the first fifty years women completed the course but did not get graduate status conferred upon them, the reasoning being, if a woman was awarded a degree it might undermine the status of the degree conferred upon the man! It was not until 1950s and 1960s that women returned to universities to collect the degrees they had completed many years before (Radio 4 Broadcast, *Woman's Hour*, 9 December 1994).

There are many people in today's mainstream education who were defined as 'ineducable' pre-1970, and denied access to an education service. These individuals were seen as the responsibility of the 'health service', only fit for 'training' and 'treatment'. It is clear that schooling systems have not learnt from their own developments and other powerful reforming movements. Our education systems have failed to understand or learn from history the consequences of their previous discriminatory practices. Such failure to learn from earlier lessons indicates that it is our schooling systems that have inherent learning difficulties and that our universities lack the wisdom to respond to the diversity within the communities in which they are supposed to serve. Universities have made many changes to open the doors but much more needs to be done. The movement towards widening participation has to go beyond its own rhetoric to create opportunities for wiser learning (DfEE, 1998). People described as having learning difficulties have a great deal to show us about how people can learn in a variety of different ways, but so far their contribution has not been considered of a 'higher order of learning' for entrance to university life. The hierarchy of learning has to change so that universities are open to learning from all members of the communities they serve.

Facilitated Communication (Biklen 1993) has provided a vehicle for many people who have for so long been denied an effective means of communication. Individuals who are discriminated against by this schooling system must find their own voice and power. There are signs of such a self-advocacy within the 'People First' movements, which are challenging the oppression of people described as having learning difficulties. This new voice will fundamentally challenge our conventional notions of communication and disability. It will force us to listen to other voices (Whittaker *et al.* 1999). Herb Lovett called such individuals 'Freedom Fighters' (Lovett 1996) and as for all such fighters they will recognise the powerful constraints and the conscious attempts to perpetuate a climate of moral intimidation where segregated special schooling is concerned. To question the status quo is seen to be 'playing politics' with 'vulnerable learners' and their families. The segregation of a learner is a highly damaging and conscious political act. The practice is one that would appear to have the tacit or overt support of people across a wide political spectrum. It is striking that members of the political left, who quite correctly struggle to eradicate racism, sexism and other barriers within our society, remain quiet at the forced segregation of people described as having learning difficulties.

In writing this chapter we do not take a neutral position on inclusive education. This would be the equivalent to taking a neutral position on racism. We believe that the present system of segregated special schools is a form of apartheid that it is equally damaging and should be repugnant to any civilised community. It has not been our intention to justify inclusion. The arguments for such a philosophy have been won. It is our intention to challenge segregated special education. We do not suggest that inclusive education is an easy option, or that it will be without struggle. We do not seek to avoid debate about the most effective strategies of support. We do not suggest that the inclusion of all learners into mainstream schools is the panacea for all our social, economic and political ills. However, with such an injustice in our present schooling system, we are corrupting the learning of all learners within it.

Factors maintaining segregation – some suggested responses

There are many powerful factors maintaining the special school system which need to be challenged, including:

- The present education legislation which is used to reject and physically segregate a learner from her/his local school and community.

What should our response be?

Working for comprehensive anti-discrimination legislation, which is enforceable, protecting the rights of all disabled and non-disabled children.

- The arbitrary assessments of the physical, social and cognitive functioning of an individual which are used to separate and isolate learners' and hence their potential for developing important relationships.

What should our response be?

Assessments and evaluations should not be used to determine a person's inclusion. If they are used they should be meaningful and carried out in a way that is understood by the individual and their family and within a context that is supportive and actively values their participation.

- Grouping certain resources together in one building and operating on the false assumption that this will meet the support requirements of all children.

What should our response be?

Resources have to be organised and arranged to meet individual requirements within the learner's locality. Training should be given to adapt or create resources that are meaningful and effective for the individual learner. We should remember that the most important resource a school has is the children within it.

- The assumption that the segregated special school has evolved over many years as the distillation of 'best practice' in supporting children with additional support requirements.

What should our response be?

We should ask 'what is "special" about special schools?'. We need to encourage good practice for every learner. What good practice has emerged from special schools continues to be tarnished because it has been applied in a limited and limiting environment. The contributions of both learners and staff are devalued by the spurious notion that they are 'special' procedures which cannot translate to mainstream settings

- That the segregated special school prepares learners for life beyond school.

What should our response be?

Most statutory 'special' educational provision for learners will end after the age of 19. Segregated special school tends to prepare learners for further segregation and generates a notion of dependency as opposed to recognition of interdependency.

- That some learners need protection from ordinary life and ordinary experiences and segregated special schools provide this.

What should our response be?

All children should have the opportunity to develop good friendships. Such relationships can provide vital lifelong supports which enable us to live ordinary, fulfilled lives. Segregated special schools restrict and in many ways prevent valuable and long-lasting relationships.

A fear of inclusion?

In addition to the practices that continue to support a segregated schooling system there are still doubts and fears expressed by some about the practicality of inclusion.

But we don't have the resources

This is often one of the most common excuses used. 'We don't have the necessary resources to teach the child who experiences learning difficulties.' If we applied the same rationale to the whole of the state schooling system we would have very few children in school. We know that very few schools have the necessary resources to meet their legal obligation to access the National Curriculum, yet they don't deny children entry to their school until they get the 'appropriate' resources.

Segregated education commands massive funding. We have to challenge the morality of using such funds to reject children and isolate them from their communities. The 'lack of resources' argument is one based upon fear rather than any serious study of the issue. The cost of including a child described as having learning difficulties is quite easily measurable, but the cost to the community of excluding the same learner from his/her community is incalculable.

But children described as having learning difficulties will be made fun of and bullied in mainstream schools

All children should be free from bullying and wherever it is experienced it has to stop. We should not assume that children are safe and protected from bullying in segregated special schools. There are many examples of abuse and bullying taking place in places of 'care'.

In a survey (Whittaker *et al.* 1999) more than a quarter of all the children who were asked 'What made them unhappy at school?' said the fear of bullying or observing bullying. Two responses were from children who said they were bullies and this made them unhappy because nobody stopped them from bullying. Again we have to look much more seriously at the factors which create the climate where bullying takes place. It is often where there is a fear of difference; and increasingly, schools and learners are expected to be the same and conform to a very narrow set of targets.

The same survey provided examples of bullying, such as name calling, being pushed out of the group by stronger children, ridiculing of family members, racist taunts, being treated unfairly, never being listened to. The same descriptions were also used to describe the actions of 'bad teachers'. Teachers and adults working in schools have an added responsibility to end bullying and stop using the behaviour on which it can be modelled. It is crucial to actively involve all young people in a process to eradicate bullying.

But we need experts to show us how to teach those individuals described as having learning difficulties

The field of learning disabilities has created a huge number of professionals who have been described as experts. We have to be suspicious of the expert; and we have to be even more suspicious of people who regard themselves as the 'experts'.

One parent remembers the birth of her child; she was quickly surrounded by a group of experts! She commented a number of years later 'They gave my child a label before I had a chance to give her a name'.

The labelling of children at birth by health experts is a cause for great concern. This initial contact and diagnosis of a child who may be said to have learning difficulties can serve to define the child and set in motion a journey to segregation and rejection for the remainder of the child's life (NWTDT 1995).

But other children will be held back by children who need lots of support

Perhaps one of the most offensive reasons for denying the access to a mainstream school for a child described as having learning difficulties is the suggestion that they may adversely affect the learning of 'others'. *All* children will affect the learning of other children they have contact with. It is that 'contact' that can be the start of important learning; it is the responsibility of the school to create positive and safe learning environments for all learners. Children are more likely to learn in environments where there is a diversity of abilities, activities and stimuli, but more significantly where they feel safe and welcome.

But what if the parents want to choose segregated special schools?

Underlying this question, asked by those advocating inclusion, is the idea that the existence of special schools could be compatible with inclusion? We have rehearsed the arguments against the provision of segregated schooling. These arguments refer to the human rights of children to be educated alongside their peers, to the fact that inclusion in the mainstream makes for good social and academic education, and that it makes good social sense in terms of reducing prejudice, stereotypes and fear of difference. The notion of parental choice does not change any of these arguments. If segregated education discriminates, then it discriminates whether chosen by parents or by the state. A full commitment to inclusion is incompatible with a view that parents can be allowed to segregate their child.

To suggest that parents are somehow outside the arguments concerning discrimination is a nonsense. Parental concerns about their children getting appropriate support, in terms of accessing the curriculum, protection from bullying, etc. can all be met through a properly resourced and organised mainstream provision, and do not require the provision of segregated schools. Rather than parents choosing special schools for their children, they could positively use their expertise and knowledge of what their child requires of a school to contribute towards developing an inclusive mainstream provision.

Parents will often 'choose' segregated special education because they believe, rightly, that they don't have a choice. Parents, like so many others, have been seduced by the myth that segregation is 'special', that the segregated school is the place where 'experts' work, and where all resources are available to meet the child's needs. However, more and more parents are recognising that they can argue for a mainstream school for their children and they are deconstructing the myth of segregated special schools (Partners in Policymaking 2001).

But the mainstream is not ready yet to accept inclusive education

For many children, mainstream schools are not working. Too often, schools are places for the adults, where children are the visitors, and where children are not listened to (Whittaker *et al.* 1999). Mainstream schools will never be creative, dynamic, safe and effective learning environments whilst they continue to discriminate against some children who learn differently and require different forms of support. Children who are at present excluded from mainstream schools are not 'the problem', they are the essence of the solution.

But how do we know if the child who experiences learning difficulties will understand what the other children are learning?

Nicholas is 16 years old and is said to have severe learning difficulties. He does not use speech; he uses a wheelchair to get around, and has some visual and hearing impairments. The school is not sure how much Nicholas is aware of his environment or how much he understands what he is taught. Should Nicholas be fully included in his local mainstream school (Elwell 2000)?

We can have Option 1

We assume Nicholas cannot understand and is not aware of his environment, so he is kept out of the mainstream school and in a segregated special school. Ten years from now we discover that we were wrong and Nicholas does understand and is very much aware of his environment. What have we lost?

Or we can have Option 2

We assume that Nicholas can understand and is aware of his environment and we fully include him in all the activities with his peers in the same classes, with appropriate supports and high expectations. Ten years from now we discover that we were wrong and that Nicholas is not aware of his environment and does not understand. What have we lost?

Towards inclusive education

One clear function special schools have always had is that they mark the limit of adult society's tolerance for children who are seen as different. These special places have become the twenty-first century gulags, where the collective fear of children who are seen as different is assuaged and their segregation from other children is reconstructed as 'special education' in a 'safe' environment. These children are, in a very real sense, the 'disappeared' young whose separation from ordinary childhood experiences and the potential for ordinary adult life is compelled by law. The segregated special school has passed its 'sell-by date'. To continue, they run the risk of participating in a practice that will come to be seen as a scandal; the separation of children from their brothers, sisters, friends and communities is increasingly recognised as inexcusable. The shifts in thinking which have influenced legislation and provision over the last forty years point the way towards an inclusive educational system. Although there is a shift in our thinking towards a more inclusive agenda, where the end to discrimination is recognised as common sense, it is unfortunately not common practice yet.

> Inclusion is expressed by terms like 'belonging', 'unity' and 'being wanted', it is not a placement it is a philosophy that says classrooms and communities are not complete unless all learners are welcome'.
>
> (Forest and O'Brien 1989)

We must continue to articulate a vision for the future. This vision is influencing the wider political structures and encouraging the growth of local mainstream schools, colleges and universities, in which every learner is actively encouraged to contribute, and where contributions are received and valued for their richness and diversity. There are many examples where inclusive education has moved beyond the rhetoric to where we can witness what is possible. It is for those who administer and those who teach to recognise that they have a responsibility to learn that different contributions can be valued equally to the benefit of all and that difference should not be sacrificed at the altar of the artificial and often arbitrary standardisation of learners.

We have to provide support that is valued as meaningful not 'Special'. In advocating such a social approach to education, we recognise that, at the present time, mainstream schools are not always organised to welcome the inclusion of all learners. Mainstream schools don't always appreciate the benefits of inclusion. Mainstream schools don't always appreciate the contributions of their existing learners. Mainstream educational systems must be improved and made more welcoming and offer more hospitality to all learners. However, regardless of the criticisms legitimately directed at the local and national organisation of some mainstream schools as they presently exist, they do have a presence and central function within the life of a local community. Such a presence can provide the scrutiny of ordinariness, which can prevent often bizarre and sometimes damaging practices adopted in segregated settings. Mainstream schools have opportunities for links to a wider community with a potential social network, enabling the learner to translate her/his presence into meaningful relationships within and beyond the school gates.

The presence of *all* learners is the first step in the eradication of irrational fears about difference – where in learning to value the contributions of others we can learn our own value.

References

Anderson, E.M. (1973) *The Disabled Schoolchild*, Buckingham, Open University.

Barnes, C. (1991) *Disabled People in Britain and Discrimination: A Case for Anti Discrimination Legislation*, London, Hurst & Company.

Biklen, D. (1992) *Schooling Without Labels*. New York, Temple University Press.

Biklen, D. (1993) *Communication Unbound*. New York, Teachers College Press.

Brandon, S. (1997) *The Invisible Wall*, published by Parents with Attitude (ISBN 0 952684 14).

Bunch, G. and Valeo, A. (1998) *Inclusion Recent Research*, Toronto, Canada, Inclusion Press.

Campbell, J. and Oliver, M. (1996) *Disabling Politics: Understanding our Past, Changing our Future*, London, Routledge.

Department of Education and Science (DES) (1978) *Special Educational Needs Report of the Committee of Inquiry into the Education of Handicapped Children and Young People* (Warnock Report), London, HMSO.

DfE (1994) *Code of Practice on: The Identification and Assessment of Special Educational Needs*, London, Central Office of Information.

DfE (1997) *Excellence for All: Meeting Special Educational Needs*, London, Central Office of Information.

DfEE (1998) *The Learning Age and Lifelong Learning*. Online: http://www. lifelonglearning.co.uk/greenpaper/index/htm

DfEE (2000) *Statistics online*: http://www.dfee.gov.uk/statistics

Department of Health (2001) *Valuing People: A New Strategy for Learning Disability for the 21st Century*. London, The Stationery Office.

Elwell, L. (2000) *Making Schools More Welcome*. Online: http://www.boltondata.org.uk/ inclusion

Finklestein, V. (2000). Here we go again, *Coalition, The Magazine of the Greater Manchester Coalition of Disabled People*, August.

Forest, M. and O'Brien, J. (1989) *Action for Inclusion*. Toronto, Inclusion Press.

Kenworthy, J. (1997) *Beyond Credit:The Funding of Segregated Education*. Bolton Data for Inclusion. Online: http://www.boltondata.org.uk/inclusion

Kenworthy, J. and Whittaker, J. (2000). Anything to declare? The struggle for inclusive education and children's rights, *Disability and Society*, 15(2): 219–231.

Lovett, H. (1996) *Learning to Listen*, London, JKP.

NorthWest Training and Development Team (NWTDT) (1995) *Breaking the News*. Online: http://www.nwtdt.u-net.com

Partners in Policymaking (2001) Contact Lynn Elwell. Online: http://www.nwtdt.u-net.com

Rae, A (1999) The Principles of Inclusive Education, *Coalition. The Magazine of the Greater Manchester Coalition of Disabled People*. August.

Salamanca (1994) *Statement and Framework for Special Education*, UNESCO Special Education Programme, 7 Place de Fontenoy, 75352 Paris 07-sp.

Thomas, F. and Ryan, J. (1987) *The Politics of Mental Handicap*. London, Free Association Press.

Tomlinson, S. (1982) *The Sociology of Special Education*, London, Routledge & Kegan Paul.

Tredgold, A.F. (1963) *Tredgold's Textbook of Mental Deficiency*, 10th edition (K. Soddy ed.), London, Baillière, Tindall and Cox.

Wade, B. and Moore, M. (1993) *Experiencing Special Education*, Milton Keynes, Open University Press.

Whittaker, J. and Crabtree, C. (1997) *How Independent are the Independent Special Needs Tribunals?* Bolton Data for Inclusion. Online: http://www.boltondata.org.uk/inclusion

Whittaker, J., Kenworthy, J. and Crabtree, C. (1999) *What Children Say about School*. Bolton Data for Inclusion. Online: http://www.boltondata.org.uk/inclusion

Chapter 5

Employment

An opportunity to belong?

Sarah Rooney

Introduction

From at least the mid-1980s it has been asserted that having a job is one of the key factors which enable people with learning difficulties to lead an 'ordinary' life. This view is not only held by academics and those individuals involved in the lives of people with learning difficulties (Warnock 1978; Wansbrough and Cooper 1980; Porterfield and Gathercole 1984; Griffiths 1989; Wertheimer 1996), but, most importantly, disabled people themselves (Kearns cited by Kennedy 1988; Atkinson and Williams 1990). Being in work is said to provide opportunities to establish and build relationships, both within and outside the workplace. It could be argued that as people with learning difficulties are frequently denied the opportunity to obtain and maintain paid employment, they have fewer chances to meet people, make friends and socialise. In short, the scarcity of work for people with learning difficulties diminishes their opportunities to belong.

Historical approaches to service provision

Before the industrialisation of work in the eighteenth and nineteenth centuries, as noted in Chapter 2 of this book, people with learning difficulties blended into their local communities. The urbanisation created by the Industrial Revolution eroded former communities and people began to be judged 'by their ability to cope with the new technological and commercial process' (Race 1995). As a result people with learning disabilities were often perceived as incompetent and unproductive. The events of this period were to have considerable impact on future generations of people with learning difficulties, as human worth was measured by work output and resulting profitability (Clapton and Fitzgerald 1998). As the nature of work changed, so did society's attitudes towards people with learning difficulties. As Race noted, and elaborated in Chapter 2:

> It was in many ways, the Industrial Revolution and the workhouse which began the isolation of people with learning disabilities from the public, and from public understanding.
>
> (Race 1995: 14)

The mechanisation of work, together with the expansion of scientific knowledge and its ensuing testing and classification of people, contributed to the development of what is now referred to as the 'medical model' of disability (Oliver 1991). Those deemed unfit to comply with the norms of a developing industrialised society were reduced to little more than a medical label and their futures were defined by a medical prognosis. It has been suggested that 'this was the era when cripples disappeared and disability was created' (Clapton and Fitzgerald 1998). Lunt and Thorton (1994) have also argued that society played a major part in creating disability and capitalism was the key in shaping the modern concept of disability. As a result, people with learning disabilities were excluded from the workplace and the communities to which they had previously belonged. New methods for controlling and accommodating economically unproductive people were established and out of the workhouse arose isolated institutions designed to segregate and contain. It has been asserted that the care of people with learning difficulties, at this time, was based upon the premise that they were a tragic burden and helplessly dependent and as such they were in need of specialised treatment and care (Ryan and Thomas 1980; Brigham 2000; Potts 2000).

Given the prevailing convictions of these times, it is difficult to imagine that the opportunity to gain open, paid employment would ever become a possibility for this marginalised group of people. However, over periods of time, services for people with learning difficulties have been exposed to shifting ideologies and changes (Oliver 1990; Malin 1995) creating new possibilities and eventual opportunities for supported living and employment.

Training for work?

Institutionalisation and segregated care dominated service provision in the first part of the twentieth century. In the 1960s, however, work-training units began to be established in hospital settings largely for the purpose of rehabilitation. The training that took place in these work units was based upon the 'readiness model', an approach founded on the belief that given sufficient training individuals might eventually develop the vocational skills that would make them employable. This process discounted the fact that in order to prepare for work, it was necessary for a person to be socially confident in addition to having experience and knowledge of employment.

Proponents of the 'readiness model' failed to recognise that many people with learning difficulties found it difficult to transfer their skills to new situations. Nor was it understood that the competencies gained within these institutional pseudo-work units had little, or no, bearing on those required within an actual workplace. The training that took place in these workshops only really served to confirm what many staff at this time believed: most of the hospital residents would not be able to cope in the outside world!

Adult training centres (ATCs) were set up in the late 1960s, by the Department of Health, to provide locally based employment training for people with learning difficulties. Their function was also to prepare people for future outside work (Barnes 1991). This approach has been referred to as the 'train and place model of vocational preparation' (Beyer and Kilsby 1996) and did not take account of the transference of skills. Many 'trainees', as day centre workers were known, became competent in craftwork, although very little preparation for other forms of employment took place. Whelan and Speake (1977) found that only 4 per cent of people undertaking work experience in adult training centres actually moved into open employment each year, although staff estimated that a possible 37 per cent were capable of paid work.

Despite this, some centres offered people the opportunity to develop expertise and engage in activities that made them feel they were skilled workers. This occurred mostly in the adult training centres that operated on the lines of sheltered industries running carpentry workshops, laundries, horticultural nurseries and sewing rooms, where toys and soft furnishing were made. 'Trainees' were often heard to speak about their pride in what they did and they referred to the adult training centre as being their place of 'work'.

Training centres began to take on sub-contract work from local manufacturers. This often took the form of simple assembly tasks and packing. The work was repetitious and monotonous and the workers were paid insultingly low wages. Zaklukiewicz (1984) has recalled with some clarity the conditions of these workshops. During the recession of the 1970s contract work became so scarce that centre managers accepted contracts for very little remuneration. This resulted in workers completing tasks for little, and in some cases, no wage at all. Many people attending adult training centres depended on contract work to keep them occupied during the day. When contracts were unavailable or terminated there was little or nothing to replace them. Contract work, and, to some extent, the craftwork that was the occupational mainstay of adult training centres, was exploitative. People were clearly not being prepared for paid employment. Neither were they being financially recompensed in an equitable way. Payment was far below the lowest wage of the day, and was often controlled by the 'instructors' staffing the day centres. Any perceived difficult or challenging behaviour that arose as a result of frustration and/or boredom incurred strict financial penalties. It was not uncommon for people to have their pay completely docked and to go home empty-handed at the end of the week.

In the early 1970s, adult training centres transferred from the Department of Health to the newly established Social Service Departments. In the same decade, the Education (Handicapped Children) Act created new optimism as the 'legal concept of ineducability' (Gray 1996: 149) was challenged. These events reflected the evolving belief that children and adults with a learning difficulty should be offered equal rights and opportunities.

In 1977 the National Development Group for the Mentally Handicapped, in its report *Day Services for Mentally Handicapped Adults* (NDG Pamphlet No. 5) recommended that a comprehensive review of adult training provision should take place. In this publication, The National Development Group (NDG), made clear recommendations about assessment procedures, record keeping, programmes, work preparation and opportunities, payment and incentives (Gray 1996). Pamphlet No 5 also promoted the concept of Social Education Centres.

Clearly the day services of this time needed transforming. Their function, still influenced by a medical model of thinking, appeared little different to that of the long-stay hospital, in that they segregated, cosseted and offered little or no scope for new opportunities and challenges (Mencap 1985).

Hindsight is a wonderful thing and it is easy to criticise the development of learning disability services over the last three decades from the safety of a new millennium. Today, it would be inconceivable for such major changes to be undertaken without at least some consultation of those who use the services. In the 1970s, however, there was no recognised mechanism for user consultation; indeed, such an idea appeared alien even to the most forward thinkers of the day.

Changing roles

As a result of the NDG's recommendations many adult training centres changed their function and ceased to offer opportunities for work. Existing provision was reviewed and new models of day service provision emerged, many providing increased opportunities for educational, social and leisure activities (Seed 1988). Some people who were affected by these changes strongly resented them as they were denied the chance to work, albeit for little or no wage.

The modification of day service provision often resulted in the more meaningful work being disbanded, with workshops and horticultural nurseries ceasing to function, whilst the more tedious contract work, which helped 'occupy' people who had no educational classes to enrol on, remained. Sheltered work enterprises were frequently replaced with 'educational' exercises that offered no more stimulation or purpose than was to be found in primary schools. Workers, who had previously spent their days making furniture became engaged in such occupations as learning to tell the time using cardboard clocks, or engaging in drama activities intended to create an awareness of road safety skills. Alternatively, groups of people with learning difficulties took part in daytime leisure activities at local swimming pools, bowling alleys and gymnasiums. These exploits, once again, reinforced stereotypical ideas of people with a learning difficulty being incapable, childlike and dependent. They also intensified ideas of segregation and difference as people with learning disabilities spent their days engaged in the recreational activities that other adults undertook in their leisure times in the evenings and at weekends (Porterfield and Gathercole 1985).

Many day centre instructors found it difficult to adapt to their newly imposed role of 'teacher'. There were few opportunities to retrain, and where they did exist they promoted quite stringent approaches to skills teaching and education. Although these approaches were grounded in the belief that people with learning disabilities could learn, the teaching programmes that were developed focused on the things people with learning difficulties were unable to do, rather than attempting to identify, and build upon, their abilities and interests. Person-centred planning and advocacies were not yet on the agenda. The individual programme plans which emerged at this time tended to reflect the views and concern of the professional and to a lesser extent the parents, rather than the individual themselves.

Supported employment: an alternative option

As adult training centres transformed into Social Education Centres, studies in America began to show that people with learning difficulties had the capacity to learn quite complex work tasks (Bellamy *et al.* 1976, 1977; Saloviita 2000). Marc Gold's (1980) *Try Another Way* approach to working with people with severe learning difficulties was considered to be innovative. This model offered more than just a systematic approach to skills teaching, as it was based upon the premise that people with learning difficulties should be shown respect, be treated with dignity, and have control over their lives. The *Try Another Way* process evolved to include training in competitive work situations and Training in Systematic Instruction developed to take on board additional factors that would enable people to work in varied workplaces.

This technology, together with the development of employment agencies in the USA resulted in the growth of supported employment schemes in Britain. These initiatives challenged the view that people with learning difficulties were unemployable (Bush 1998).

The changes to day centre provision ran parallel with the escalating closures of long-stay hospitals. This resulted in day services providing a variety of educational, social and leisure activities to people drawn from wide ability and age ranges. Given this diversity, it was unlikely that all those seeking vocational training and/or work placement would have their needs met. The Independent Development Council (1984) recognised that day services had an 'almost impossible role to play ... which resulted in no single function being performed adequately'. The supported employment model was developed in an attempt to address this deficiency in service provision. Mencap's Pathway Employment Project, created in the mid-1970s, was one such response. Other supported employment initiatives such as the Shaw Trust and Blakes Warfe employment service followed in the mid-1980s. They strove to challenge the 'readiness model' by exploring ways of placing people with learning difficulties directly into paid employment (Ashton 1995).

The generic term 'supported employment' encompasses several different work models such as enclaves, mobile work crews, sheltered workshops and workers' co-operatives (Lutfiyya *et al.* 1988). The definition of supported employment, as understood by most supported employment agencies in Britain today, however, is the placing of individuals with a learning disability directly into competitive employment (Beyer *et al.* 1996; Wertheimer, 1996). This is sometimes referred to as the 'place, train and maintain' model. Supported employment workers or job coaches offer a time-limited service to the individual seeking work. This includes help locating a job for the person and then providing one-to-one on-site employment-based training. Unlike previous development programmes the supported employment process begins with individual vocational assessment and profiling, completed prior to a person being found work. The assessment profile is designed to gain an understanding of a person's employment aspirations and capabilities and their strengths and limitations, thus providing insight into their support needs. The vocational profile uses this information to identify a suitable job. It is also used to record any practical arrangements such as benefits and transport that affect a person's availability and ability to work. Although job coaches provide individually tailored support, they 'fade away' once the person can work independently or when a 'co-worker' has been enlisted to undertake 'in-house' mentoring. This method of working represents a real transformation in the way people with learning difficulties are supported to spend their days. As a result increasing numbers of people are being encouraged to work in their local communities once again.

A personal perspective

A gradual change in public attitude, together with the development of person-centred employment services and more enlightened social care policy has led to increased work opportunities for people with learning difficulties (DfEE 1996). Despite these important developments, the question still remains: does having a job address the wrongs of the past and enable people with learning difficulties to take their place in society? Do they, in fact, really belong? To help with answering this question, twelve people with learning difficulties, who have gained employment through a supported employment service, agreed to take part in discussions that focused on their relationships in work and their social opportunities within their local communities. This was the 'What about the Workers' support group, which is affiliated to a supported employment service, in Oldham. The group meets once a month to discuss employment related issues and members take part in requested training activities. Guest speakers are invited to talk about new or different social activities that people can become involved in. The group members said that they value the opportunity to meet together in a less formal way as well, and organise at least one additional social outing a month.

The 'workers' commented that the support group offered the opportunity to get together 'to make friends, meet people and arrange what you are going to do'. Meetings enable them to 'talk about what is going on in work' and to maintain links with the employment service once one-to-one support in the workplace is no longer needed. Although only a few individuals got together outside of the monthly meeting and social events, the group members stated that the gatherings meant they could 'socialise, see each other, have company and discuss any problems'. Social outings varied from a trip to Blackpool, to a meal out, or simply going to the pub together. Two women opined that they 'would miss [the group] it if it wasn't there' and that the meetings represented one of the few opportunities they had to get out and be with people in the evenings. 'If the workers' group wasn't here I'd just sit at home in the evening, because it's not safe to go out at night.' Many of the 'workers' also attended Gateway Clubs, specialised church-organised learning disability 'youth groups' and segregated swimming clubs. Other out of work periods of the week were spent with family at home.

All the people in the group work, although not all have full-time paid employment. Some have part-time employment because, in spite of the availability of Disability Tax Credits, and Disability-Working Allowances, they were concerned about losing their benefits, or that their earnings would not provide a decent basic income. Two people worked in Sheltered Workshops, one person undertook unpaid work, but reported that she was happy with this situation. None of the individuals received job coach support any longer. Group members were employed in various settings such as offices, factories, shops and the local theatre. The actual roles undertaken within these employment environments were also diverse. One person constructed complex electronic circuit boards, one was a porter in a pharmaceutical company, while another worked in the company canteen. All group members were employed in busy workplaces surrounded by colleagues.

Without exception, everyone said that they enjoyed their job. They reported: 'It keeps me busy and off the streets more than anything'; 'It's something to do, rather than sitting at home doing nothing'; 'I like getting out and getting involved'; 'It keeps me occupied, it's better than sitting around in the day centre'; 'So you are not in the house all the time, I'm not getting into mischief'; 'It's a bit more challenging, a bit different 'cos you are working with ordinary people'; 'Going out and about; it gives you satisfaction, I'd like to be working all the time'; 'I like everything about work, it makes me really happy to do anything they throw at me'; 'I like helping out and getting involved'.

Although some 'workers' commented on minor irritations related to the job they did, such as 'confusion, feeling uncomfortable when there's a new job' or 'not liking welding' or being frustrated when the photocopier broke down, all were positive about being in work. Employment provided them with stimulation, challenges, new opportunities and the chance to do something more meaningful than walking the streets, sitting at home or attending a day centre. This applied equally to all work situations, even to those who were unpaid. However, for those who had full-time paid employment money was clearly an important incentive. A wage enabled them to pay for commodities such as clothes, CDs and videos. Having spending power meant that these people were able to enjoy ordinary everyday activities like shopping, which provided a focus for the weekend, and a topic of conversation for Monday morning. Having more money in their pocket, in theory, created opportunities for an evening's entertainment in the pub or meant they could afford to visit the cinema, although in practice only one person actually did these things.

Being in work provided a natural setting for meeting people, although this, of course, depended on the type of job undertaken. The 'workers' all had employment that enabled them to be with other people, even though for some this occurred within a segregated sheltered environment. Those who spent their days in ordinary work settings commented on their opportunity to meet and talk to a variety of people. One person said that 'I've worked with disabled people, 'cos I'm a disabled person, but lots of people would prefer working with both – I'm the sort of person who would get on with anyone.' Another commented that 'it was nice to talk to different people'.

The 'workers' said that they chatted to their work colleagues, and all but one reported that their colleagues were friendly, helpful and approachable. 'I talk to me workmates – there's some nice people I work with'. One person had unfortunately experienced victimisation in the workplace, which resulted in him changing his job. The opportunity to talk to colleagues varied according to the job undertaken. For some, conversation occurred naturally as they worked together. Those who worked in busy workshops waited until dinner and break times to chat. Others involved in the service or retail industry said they appreciated the chance to talk to customers as well as other members of the staff.

Having a job presents opportunities to meet a wider mix of people than spending time in segregated day services or sheltered workshops. It does not, however, for this particular group appear to encourage them to meet and socialise with their colleagues out of the work situation. A few said that they would go to the annual Christmas party, or meal, but would not get involved in anything else. There were several reasons for this. Travelling alone at night and feeling vulnerable in an inner-city area was a frequent concern. Some were unable to travel independently and saw this as a barrier to mixing with colleagues away from work. They felt that they could not impose by asking for a lift and were embarrassed by the fact they could not drive or travel on their own to evening functions. People said they were asked to go on work outings, but they felt that although colleagues asked them to join them at evening and weekend events, they 'don't talk to us if we go out – they leave us out'. One person said that he needed to join the sports and social welfare club first and he 'hadn't bothered to do it'. Only one person said that he met people from work for a drink in the evening, but that this was not on a regular weekly basis.

Conclusions

The aim of this chapter was to reflect upon the history and development of employment opportunities for people with learning difficulties. It also sought to examine whether the increased opportunities for work outside of day centre provision in recent times enable people with learning difficulties to establish and develop a wider network of relationships.

All of us meet, and develop friendship networks in different ways. This can be through families and neighbours, by maintaining old friendships from school and through leisure and community activities, as well as through work. Although having a job opens up possibilities for relationships, not everyone chooses to socialise with colleagues outside of work. Indeed, many people are surprised to discover how little they actually have in common when they meet in different environments and circumstances. Work might provide the only link and for relationships closer than that of acquaintance to flourish, this may simply be not enough. Sociologists (Haralambos and Holborn 1991) have argued that in contemporary society many people lead private and home-centred existences. Social life is frequently spent watching television, playing computer games, communicating via the Internet, doing work around the home or spending time with one's family. Despite this, work plays an important role in the lives of most people. It defines who we are, offers opportunities for enrichment and self-improvement and, at the very least, provides a reason to get out of bed in the morning.

If the above is true for the majority, then the 'workers' group experience of employment is not so very different. Although having a job was clearly important to them, many spent much of their leisure time at home. However, their comments regarding the 'workers' group seemed to indicate that they needed more than just home-based leisure, possibly because work in itself did not totally fulfil their need for companionship and friendship.

Clearly work offers these people opportunities for inclusion. Each person who took part in the discussions had positive comments to make about the people they worked with. Work was an important part of their lives, even for those who worked within sheltered workshops, and was valued more highly than spending time at a day centre, or at home. Many commented upon the importance of contributing and spending their day in purposeful activity. Most of the 'workers' felt accepted by work colleagues. There were natural opportunities to come together and talk in the day, even though these relationships did not particularly extend to out of work activities

It was evident, however, that work is not a panacea for loneliness, or a guarantee of companionship. In fact, having the opportunity to extend their relationship networks and observe other lifestyles more closely seemed to highlight relationship gaps that occur in their lives. As one of the workers wryly commented 'I would go to the socials if I had someone to go with – they all go with their husbands'.

Part-time employment was also seen as a barrier to making closer relationships. 'I work with different people on different days, so I don't get to know them very well.' This lack of continuity may pose a problem for all part-time employees, but may be particularly difficult for those workers with learning difficulties, who lack the social skills or confidence needed to create and maintain relationships (Beyer et al. 1995). Studies by Lister et al. (1992) and O'Bryan et al. (2000) have also indicated this problem is far from unique, as a high percentage of people with learning difficulties who work do so on a part-time basis, notably sixteen hours or less a week. The part-time/full-time debate is important as it clearly affects a person's ability to make connections. Kilsby et al. (1995) and Mank et al. (1999) drew similar conclusions. Their research indicated that people with learning difficulties achieve better integration in the work place if their weekly hours and work schedules match that of their fellow employers.

O'Bryan et al.'s (2000) research has stressed that social security benefits represent a major obstacle to securing full-time employment. Their observations were commensurate with the experience of some of the 'workers'. The complexities of understanding, and managing the benefit system, was a major consideration for both the individual and their family. Often a 'worker's' comments appeared to reflect parental concerns of 'what will happen if I lose my benefits'. This remains a formidable barrier to many people with learning difficulties seeking full-time employment and thus developing wider relationships through work. This issue needs addressing if people with learning difficulties are to be included through having a job. As Simons and Watson (1999) have argued, although 'work might have a useful role in opening social networks, the current framework effectively minimises that possibility' (p. 58).

Despite the fact that they did not meet colleagues after work, the 'workers' indicated that having a job was generally worth while in terms of extending their social relationships. They had the opportunity to work alongside a number of different people. The relationship formed through work tended to be that of 'acquaintance' rather than friend. Typically most people have a mixture of connections in their lives. It is, however, relatively new for many people with learning difficulties to have the opportunity to expand their networks so that they include even acquaintances. People who previously lived and/or worked in institutions and day centres had limited experience of being part of a wider community. Having a job, at the very least, offers the opportunities to participate in everyday activities, with local people.

These opportunities, as valuable as they are, do not enable the 'workers' to completely overcome their feelings of loneliness and exclusion or, at times, their sense of social failure. Indeed, sometimes these appeared prominent, and two individuals were acutely aware of their lack of a partner to take to social functions, while others were embarrassed at being unable to travel independently and of their vulnerability when out alone at night.

Although it could be argued that improvement in the quality of life of people with learning difficulties depends upon their wider participation in 'ordinary' activities, and settings, no one should be prescriptive about who people spend time with. The concept of friendship is complex and operates on different levels. Friends might simply provide company, or be people in whom we can confide, who have an understanding of our life experiences (Firth and Rapley 1990; Richardson and Ritchie 1990).

The creation of the 'workers' group resulted from a requirement stipulated in the Supported Employment Service's bid for European Social Funding, and it is clear that it fulfils an important function. The people with learning difficulties who took part in this research appreciate the opportunity to belong to a group that is flexible enough to offer different types of assistance. The 'workers' group provides companionship and advice, has a social component, and also acts as a 'self-help' group. These meetings provide the opportunity to relax, meet up with old friends from the day centres, and form a circle of support in which they can discuss work-related concerns in a 'safe' arena. The group also provides opportunities for self-development and determination through the acquisition of self-advocacy and leadership skills.

A member of the supported employment service facilitates the group. The service it offers, however, could be perceived by some as being a step backwards. Judgements are frequently made about the social status accorded to groupings of so-called 'devalued' people and it is possible that this group might be criticised for encouraging an association which perpetuates a 'segregated position in a "handicapped world"' (Chappell 1994: 424).

Alternatively, these relationships might be seen to represent much more. People in power have for so long defined the living, working and social circumstances of people with learning difficulties. Their past and to some extent their future, have been influenced by prevailing 'professional' ideologies which have, at various moments in time, chosen to 'include' or 'exclude' them from both their wider and local communities. Great emphasis is now placed upon people with learning disabilities accessing ordinary opportunities through supported employment, natural supports and individualised paid assistance via Direct Payments. Although these developments are in many ways admirable, it is important that we recognise that total integration may lead to some people being dispersed into a world that is not always friendly, secure or welcoming. Chappell (1994: 426), concerned about this issue, has suggested that disabled people run the risk of being isolated, both 'physically and emotionally in a non-disabled community'. Lindsey (2001: 11) has argued that 'assimilation [into mainstream workplaces] can be progression into isolation'. The Department of Health also commented on this issue in their report *Facing the Facts* (1999: 17) when they observed 'people with learning disabilities in paid employment have difficulty building up a social life as this did not arise from work relationships'. A study by Bass and Drewett (1997) has also indicated that relationships with colleagues did not extend beyond the workplace.

The importance of facilitating the kind of support that the 'workers' group provides should not be ignored. People choose to attend the monthly meetings and other social events; they are not required to. Some of them meet together outside of these gatherings. Similarly many of the 'workers' chose to go to other segregated evening clubs such as Gateway Clubs. It could, however, be argued that they 'hang on' to this type of provision because they are not yet accustomed or confident enough to enjoy more 'mainstream' social events.

All group members have their own reasons for attending the 'workers group', whether it be for friendship, social identity or because the group operates within a safe and secure environment. One thing, however, is clear. People should not be 'signed off' once they have left day services and moved into employment. Many will need the security of knowing there is some point of reference to which they can return. The relaxed, social format of the 'workers group' makes it easy to keep in touch. Contacting their employment worker, once their one-to-one job coach role is over may lower a person's self-esteem as they may feel because they still require some support that others will perceive they have 'failed'. Additionally, staff working within supported employment agencies carry heavy 'case-loads' and it is impossible to maintain contact on a regular basis with all those who are in work. Even when the 'workers' do not have problems to discuss, it is important for them to know that they can share their successes with those who truly understand how far they have travelled in not only obtaining employment, but successfully maintaining it as well.

Equally a person with a learning difficulty may need to have an organisation or group to 'hang on to', in the same way that other people return to groups that have been important at some point in their lives, such as the reunions of old school friends. The 'workers group' may fulfil such a function, by providing the opportunity for a group of people with learning difficulties, who share similar histories and experiences, to meet together. This could be crucial in the future, when parents are no longer alive and retirement from work looms close, and learning disability services have other priorities. This group is not the 'sum total' of who the members are. It does not try to prescribe where the 'workers' live, work or play or who they see. It does not define who they are. It exists simply to offer a listening ear, advice and companionship.

Employment is clearly on the Government's agenda for the twenty-first century. This represents a huge ideological shift from the reasoning of a hundred years ago when people with learning difficulties were perceived as 'defective' and 'inadequate'. Objective eight of the DoH (2001) White Paper *Valuing People*, states the Government's intention:

> To enable more people with learning disabilities to participate in all forms of employment, wherever possible in paid work and to make a valued contribution to the world of work.
>
> (p. 81)

This will be achieved by a number of 'key action points':

- New targets for the number of people with learning difficulties in work.
- Renaming of the Government Supported Employment Programme to 'Work-step', which will focus on helping disabled people move into mainstream employment.
- Amalgamation of the Employment Service and Benefits Agency, to be known as the 'Working Age Agency', creating a forum to look at the way benefits affect the opportunity to work.
- Development of the New Deal for Disabled People (NDDP) and a network of job brokers, who will have the skills to work with people with learning difficulties.
- Better employment opportunities within the Public Sector, and target setting for Local Councils for the employment of socially excluded people, as part of Local Public Service Agreements.
- Welfare to Work Joint Investment Plans to be in place from April 2001 onwards.
- Local Employment Services to be members of the Learning Disability Partnership Boards.

These are, of course, excellent initiatives, which will, hopefully, lead to greater numbers of people with learning difficulties becoming employed. It is important for those in positions of power to remember that although predetermined performance indicators and outcomes have been achieved, and people with learning difficulties get jobs, they should not be deserted. Employment is no guarantee of friendship and bullying is no stranger to the workplace. A King's Fund briefing paper (1999: 2) made the following observations:

> A history of segregation has left communities without the skills to communicate with people with learning disabilities. Much has been learnt about how to support people to develop social networks and participate in the activities of the rest of the community but progress is slow and only the minority are successful.

It is, therefore, crucial that a local level 'fallback' strategy resembling the 'What about the Workers Group' exists to try and ensure that people's social and emotional needs, which may not always be met through work, are not forgotten. If we assume that having a job will be all things to all people, we run the risk of many people with learning difficulties becoming isolated once again, by abandoning them within a community that does not always care.

References

Ashton, D. (1995) *Survey of Supported Employment in the Northwest*, Whalley, Northwest Training and Development Team.

Atkinson, D. and Williams, F. (1990) *Know Me as I Am. An Anthology of Prose, Poetry and Art by People with Learning Difficulties*, London, Hodder and Stoughton.

Barnes, C. (1991) *Disabled People in Britain: A Case for Anti-discriminatory Legislation*, London, University of Calgary Press.

Bass, M. and Drewett, R. (1997) *Real Work: Supported Employment for People with Learning Difficulties*, Sheffield, Joint Unit for Social Services Research, Sheffield University.

Bellamy, G.T., Horner, R.H. and Inman, D.P. (1976) *Habilitation of Severely and Profoundly Retarded Adults: Reports from the Specialised Training Programme* (Vol. 1), Eugene, University of Oregon.

Bellamy, G.T., Horner, R.H. and Inman, D.P. (1977) *Habilitation of Severely and Profoundly Retarded Adults: Reports from the Specialised Training Programme* (Vol. 2), Eugene, University of Oregon.

Beyer, S. and Kilsby, M. (1996) *The Costs and Benefits of Supported Employment Agencies*, Cardiff, Welsh Centre for Learning Disabilities, Applied Research Unit.

Beyer, S., Kilsby, M. and Willson, C. (1995) Interaction and engagement of workers in supported employment: a British comparison between workers with and without learning disabilities, *Mental Handicap Research*, 8(3): 137–154.

Beyer, S., Goodere, L. and Kilsby, M. (1996) *The Cost and Benefits of Supported Employment Agencies*, Cardiff, Welsh Centre for Learning Disabilities, Applied Research Unit.

Brigham, L. (2000) Understanding segregation from the nineteenth to the twentieth century: redrawing the boundaries and the problems of 'pollution'. In: L. Brigham, D. Atkinson,

M. Jackson, S. Rolph and J. Walmsley, *Crossing Boundaries. Change and Continuity in the History of Learning Disability Services*, Kidderminster, BILD.

Bush, T. (1998) Ready, willing and waiting: supporting employment and people with learning disabilities, *Journal of Learning Disabilities for Nursing, Health and Social Care*, 2(4): 221–224.

Chappell, A. (1994) A question of friendship: community care and the relationship of people with learning difficulties, *Disability and Society*, 9(4): 419–433.

Clapton, J. and Fitzgerald, J. (1998) The History of Disability: A History of 'Otherness', *New Renaissance Magazine*, 7(1): 32–43.

DfEE (1996) *Disability Discrimination Act 1995: What employers needs to know*, London, HMSO.

Department of Health (1999) *Facing the Facts: Services for People with Learning Disabilities*, Policy Impact Study of Social Care and Health Studies, London, The Stationery Office.

Department of Health (2001) *Valuing People. A New Strategy for Learning Disability for the 21st Century*, London, The Stationery Office.

Firth, H. and Rapley, M. (1990) *From Acquaintance to Friendship: Issues for People with Learning Disabilities*, Kidderminster, British Institute of Mental Handicap.

Gold, M. (1980) *Try Another Way Training Manual*, Champaign, IL, Research Press.

Gray, G. (1996) Changing day services. In: P. Mittler and V. Sinason, *Changing Policy and Practice for People with Learning Disabilities*, London, Cassell Education.

Griffiths, M. (1989) *Enabled to Work: Support into Employment for Young People with Disabilities*, London, Further Education Unit.

Haralambos, M. and Holborn, M. (1991) *Sociology. Themes and Perspective*, 3rd edition, London, Collins.

Independent Development Council for People with Mental Handicap (1984) *Next Steps*, London, King's Fund Centre.

Kennedy, M. (1988) *From Sheltered Workshops to Supported Employment*, Center on Human Policy, Syracuse University.

Kilsby, M., Beyer, S. and Evans, S. (1995) Supported employment and interaction: a full-time or part-time service?, *Lias*, 36: 9–12

King's Fund (1999) *Learning Disabilities: From care to citizenship*, Briefing Paper No. 4, London, King's Fund Centre.

Lindsey, E. (2001) Willing and able, *Guardian Society*, 10 January: 2–3.

Lister, T., Ellis, L., Phillips, T., O'Bryan, A., Beyer, S. and Kilsby, M. (1992) *Survey of Supported Employment Services in England, Scotland and Wales*, Manchester, National Development Team.

Lunt, N. and Thorton, P. (1994) Disability and employment: towards an understanding of discourse and policy, *Disability & Society*, 9(2): 223–239.

Lutfiyya, Z., Rogan, P. and Shoultz, B. (1988) *Supported Employment: A Conceptual Overview*, Syracuse, Centre on Human Policy Research and Training Centre on Community Integration, Syracuse University.

Malin, N. (1995) *Services for People with Learning Disabilities*, London: Routledge.

Mank, D., Cioffi, A. and Yovanoff, P (1999) Impact of coworkers' involvement with supported employees on wage and integration outcomes, *Mental Retardation*. 37(5): 383–394.

Mencap (1985) *Day Services Today and Tomorrow: Mencap's vision of Daytime Services for People with Mental Handicap.* London, Mencap.

National Development Group (NDG) (1977) *Pamphlet No. 5: Day Services for Mentally Handicapped Adults*, London, HMSO.

O'Bryan, A., Simons, K., Beyer, S. and Grove, B. (2000) *A Framework for Supported Employment*, York, Joseph Roundtree Foundation.

Oliver, M. (1990) *The Politics of Disablement*, London, Macmillan.

Oliver, M. (1991) Disability and participation in the labour market. In: P. Brown and R. Scase (eds) *Poor Work: Disadvantage and the Division of Labour*. Buckingham, Open University Press, pp.132–146.

Porterfield, J. and Gathercole, C. (1984) *The Employment of People with a Mental Handicap: Progress Towards an Ordinary Working Life*, London, King's Fund Centre.

Potts, P. (2000) Concrete representation of a social category: consolidating and transforming public institutions for people classified as 'defective.' In L. Brigham, D. Atkinson, M. Jackson, S. Rolph and J. Walmsley, *Crossing Boundaries. Change and Continuity in the History of Learning Disability Services*, Kidderminster, BILD.

Race, D. (1995) Historical development of service provision. In: N. Malin, *Services for People with Learning Disabilities*, London, Routledge.

Richardson, A. and Ritchie, J. (1990) Developing friendships. In: T. Booth (ed.) *Better Lives: Changing Services for People with Learning Difficulties*, Social Services Monographs, Research in Practice, Joint Unit for Social Services Research, University of Sheffield.

Ryan, J. and Thomas, F. (1980) *The Politics of Mental Handicap*, Harmondsworth, Penguin Books.

Saloviita, T. (2000) Supported employment as a paradigm shift and a cause of legitimation crisis, *Disability & Society*, 15(1): 87–98.

Seed, P. (1988) *Day Care at the Crossroads*, Tunbridge, Costello.

Simons, K. and Watson, D. (1999) *The View from Arthurs' Seat. A Literature Review of Housing and Support Options 'Beyond Scotland'*, Edinburgh, Scottish Executive.

Wansbrough, N. and Cooper, P. (1980) *Open Employment after Mental Illness*, London, Tavistock Publications.

Warnock, M. (1978) *Special Educational Needs: Report of a Committee of Enquiry into the Education of Handicapped Children and Young People*, The Warnock Report, London, HMSO.

Wertheimer, A. (ed.) (1996) *Changing Days. Developing New Day Opportunities with People who have Learning Difficulties*, London, King's Fund.

Whelan, E. and Speake, B. (1977) *Adult Training Centres in England and Wales*. Manchester, National Association of Teachers of the Mentally Handicapped.

Zaklukiewicz, S. (1984) *Development in Day Care*, Edinburgh, Scottish Council for Research in Education.

Chapter 6

Management and change

David Race

Introduction

From the thesis of the same naive researcher whose conclusions on the learning disability scene of the 1970s began Chapter 2 came the proposition of a 'new service for the mentally handicapped' based on ordinary housing and, more importantly for the subject of this chapter, based on one Local Authority organisation for learning disability services. In introducing this idea, I noted that:

> Recommending a combined service is not new, with such writers as Tizard (1974), Thomas (1973) and Blunden (1975) proposing jointly planned facilities or a new profession. None of these writers, however, discusses fully the organisation which might be conducive to producing an efficient integrated service.
>
> (Race 1977: 209)

I also remarked that the Jay Committee, who were sitting as that thesis was completed, might be considering similar reorganisation, but cautioned that history suggested that such a radical step was unlikely, even with the weight of a governmental committee. Such proved to be the case; the Jay Committee did not recommend organisational change, but a combined profession with a common training. Chapter 2 notes, too, that some of the reasons why even that proposal was dropped had much to do with organisational power within the NHS. At the time I noted, as had others (Rowbottom 1973), that the longer standing national hierarchy and professional status of the NHS tended to produce an assumption of dominance over the fledgling Local Authority Social Services Departments.

Moving forward twenty-five years, again with some sense of *déjà vu*, this chapter argues that changes in the organisation and finances of learning disability services, as part of wider changes in government structures and the redefinition of the welfare state, have altered who pays for, plans, and, most dramatically, who provides those services. What has altered less, however, is the impact of those services on the people who use them. The organisational aspects of the community care changes of the 1980s and 1990s will be analysed in this way, as will the New Labour

Government's 'modernisation programme' for services and its White Paper *Valuing People* (DoH 2001). We begin, however, with the creation of Social Services Departments.

Organisations and services – the new Social Services Departments

A great many of the organisational arrangements examined in this chapter are not specifically related to learning disability, but to larger organisational developments in the service world of which learning disability is only a small part. Taking the NHS first, organisational arrangements, in the twenty or more years between its inception and the publication of the Seebohm Report (Home Office *et al.* 1968) had seen some changes, and the early 1970s were to see some more. The fundamental structure, however, of a hierarchical organisation, financed centrally through the Department of Health and Social Security (DHSS), with regional and more locally based administrative bodies, was unchanged. In this respect locally elected representatives, whilst they served as part of hospital and health authority boards, took their place alongside appointed members not answerable to any set of voters. Planning could thus take place centrally and regionally, ensuring a degree of consistency and control over local policies (Rowbottom 1973).

Local Authorities, on the other hand, were and are controlled by elected and at least theoretically accountable councillors, with powers to vary their finances through the setting of local property taxes (known then as 'rates'). Though they still relied on substantial funding from central government in the form of the 'rate support grant', the power of local councils to determine priorities in spending were considerable, especially in the big departments of Housing and Education. When Seebohm recommended a 'one door' Local Authority department, to address all the social welfare needs of its population, the stage was set for an expansion of the fairly small Children's Departments and even smaller Welfare Departments into Social Services Departments that would take up a substantial portion of the local authority resource cake.

As they began, in 1973, to feel their way into some form of organisational structure, Social Services Departments also began to feel their way into the sorts of services they might provide for different 'client groups', as the language of the time would put it. Those within the new organisations with a background in learning disability were relatively few, and rarely among the new Directors and Assistant Directors. There was thus little political power and knowledge within the new departments for learning disability services to take advantage of the external power felt from the White Paper *Better Services for the Mentally Handicapped* (DHSS 1971) and its accompanying capital finance.

What did this mean in terms of an effect on the development of services? To attempt to answer this question, we need to look in a little more detail at the sort of organisational structures that emerged in the new Social Services. Two main structures seem to have evolved. In the first, Brunel University's Research Unit

(BIOSS), in their major study (Rowbottom 1974), divided the organisation between the two main functions of service, broadly defined as 'residential' and 'day care', while the other first divided the organisation into geographic regions, and then, for each region, split organisationally between residential and day care. Since these structures were to remain largely unchanged for the next twenty years we can look at the management of learning disability services within them, in order to fully appreciate the impact of later developments.

The place of Social Services Departments within Local Authority structures should also be borne in mind here. Like other departments of the authority their ultimate controlling body was the full council, made up of the elected members of the various constituencies of the authority. For ease of administration, however, day-to-day power rested with a series of committees and sub-committees, reflecting the political balance of the parties on the full council. Officers of the departments therefore reported to their respective committees and sub-committees. In the case of Social Services the Director would report to the full Social Services Committee (and occasionally to the full council) and, together with or represented by Assistant Directors, to sub-committees such as finance or planning. Proposals for services, especially new services, would thus be very much in the hands of the second- and third-tier management, the Assistant Directors and specialist managers.

Looking at BIOSS's two models shows how power over service development was likely to be in the hands of non-specialists, as far as learning disability was concerned. In the 'Functional Model' learning disability services would usually be split between residential and day care, with an Assistant Director for Residential Care having hostels, often for both adults and children, under their remit, along with 'homes' for other client groups. A specialist in learning disability at third-tier level would again be relatively rare, most being ex 'mental welfare officers', who had responsibility for general 'mental health clients' as well as people with learning difficulties. Parents or others seeking residential services would therefore be referred by the 'field' social worker, either to individual hostels, or to the third-tier manager, and decisions on admission would be in their hands, usually based on availability of places and the perceived 'social competence' of the individual concerned. If they were considered unsuitable, then admission to the local (or at least the nearest) hospital would be sought, with admission depending almost entirely on the decision of the consultant psychiatrist. In both cases, of course, the organisation deciding on the 'need', i.e. the service that a person required, would be the same as that providing the service, and needs assessments were often referred to in terms, for example, of someone being 'in need of a hostel' or 'in need of a hospital' rather than being 'in need of somewhere to live'. On the whole, therefore, unless particular individuals within the organisation were up to date with the rapidly changing learning disability debates of the 1970s, Social Services Departments would tend to operate in a reactive way, led by national policy and finance, based on the assumptions of the DHSS, itself totally dominated at advisory level by nurses and doctors.

This would be still more the case in the 'Geographical Model' described by BIOSS. If the chances of a learning disability specialist at senior level in the functional organisation were low, still more so would be the situation in the geographical form, which specialised one tier lower. Geographical second-tier managers would have responsibility for all services, with the residential/day service split at third tier, and specialism by client group below that, although some authorities split by client group below the regional manager. Either way, all client groups came under one individual regional manager, who would tend to act some-what more as an administrator of fairly autonomous residential and day service units. Managers of these units, for learning disability almost totally either hostels or adult training centres, would not often, in the early 1970s, have a background in learning disability, but come from residential services for elderly people or children, or, in the case of adult training centres, from an industrial background.

As resources, and therefore some degree of power, rose in the 1970s for learning disability services, so too did calls for more training for staff, especially senior staff. In keeping with the 'generic' spirit of Seebohm, however, qualifications available to managers of hostels or day centres were either the generic Certificate of Qualification in Social Work (CQSW) or a generic Certificate of Social Service (introduced in 1977). Some Social Services Departments, faced with the absence of specialists in 'mental handicap', looked to qualified nurses (usually with the 'Registered Nurse Mental Subnormality' qualification) to run their hostels. When this lack of specialists is set alongside the radical debates of the 1970s, first over 'hostels versus hospitals' (Shapiro 1974; Elliot 1975), then over the role of adult training centres, following 'Pamphlet Five' from the National Development Group in 1977 with its call for 'Social Education Centres' (see Chapters 2 and 5), it is not surprising that calls for a unified service, such as those discussed in the introduction, were made. The difficulty was, as noted above, that only a very small voice for learning disability existed at senior levels in Social Services Departments, and co-ordination with Health Authorities was very tenuous. More formal mechanisms were tried within service structures, such as what was known as 'joint finance', money made available to take people out of hospital, but this again tended to operate at the margins of both health and social services budgets. Much faith was therefore put in the Jay Committee in trying to provide some credibility for joint working, but, as we have seen in Chapter 2, the incoming government quietly buried their report, leaving the respective organisational structures essentially unchanged. What that government was also to bring, however, and what was to have a much greater effect on the organisation and financing of services, was the arrival of the 'quasi-market' (Le Grand 1990) in public services.

The quasi-market cometh – changes in the 1980s

The new Thatcher Government inherited an organisational structure, namely Health Authorities and Social Services Departments, that controlled and provided the vast bulk of learning disability services in any given locality (though an exact match of geographical boundaries was rare). The fact that there were considerable variations in the budgets of these two organisations, and between them and their geographical neighbours, meant that the resources allocated to specific groups would also vary markedly.

Additionally, of course, Local Authorities were, and are, political organisations, and at the start of the 1980s local politicians also formed part of the membership of Health Authorities. This meant that political activity was central to decision making about policy and the allocation of resources. So not only was power concentrated in a few local organisations, but political loyalties, such as those between local Labour parties and the public service unions, or Conservatives and local businesses, including those involved in the construction of 'public works', would all play their part in decisions affecting services for individuals and families. The knowledge of any of these people, either professionals or politicians, of learning disability issues was thus not likely to be very deep, and even where it existed, it would play a minor role in comparison to the other considerations of the complex political and administrative system of which they were a part.

A major new element then entered the equation, initially in services with more obvious equivalents in the marketplace, such as waste disposal or catering, but then extending to the whole gamut of public provision. This was the notion of services as 'commodities' which could be subject to the 'disciplines of the market'. The ideological commitment to 'neo-classical' economics of the so-called 'new right' of Thatcherism produced a powerful critique of the Welfare State. Public agencies, especially Local Authorities, were seen as being 'protected from competitive forces and thereby the necessary spurs to efficiency that the market provides' (Wistow et al. 1994)

Especially in the second and third Thatcher terms, following the defeat of the miners, increasingly powerful union legislation, and a booming economy for those in employment, the 'success' of market-driven policies began to be felt in the services sector. For learning disability services this was most directly encountered in the general developments on 'community care' leading to the NHS and Community Care Act of 1990, and these will be discussed later. Before that, however, consideration needs to be given to contemporary developments in the financing of services, whose interaction with the organisational issues mentioned above proved the determining factor in the final shape of the legislation.

The colour of money – the power of resources over the shape of services

It was something of a badge of honour of the Thatcher Government to be reducing 'public spending', thereby freeing 'taxpayers' money' to be returned to them in the form of tax cuts. On the other hand, expenditure on politically popular services, especially the NHS, was claimed to be rapidly rising, with the NHS being famously 'safe in our hands'. What also characterised this debate was the developing antagonism, especially as local elections returned more and more non-Conservative councillors, between local and central government. Thus the central government could impose, via a device called the Standard Spending Assessment (SSA) a crude notion of what Local Authorities should be spending, and back this up with a central judgement of the levels of grant from the centre, whilst at the same time 'capping' Local Authorities who sought to offset the loss of central revenue by raising the local rates. In addition, central government already had total control over monetary payments to individuals through the social security system, and over expenditure on the NHS, even removing the partial representation on regional and area health authorities of elected councillors, making them totally appointed bodies. As noted by various commentators (Hutton 1996), the way in which this power was used led to greater and greater 'centralisation' of decision making. The effect of this was to produce some confusing sets of statistics on what could be called 'welfare spending' as the 1980s progressed. While overall figures suggested an increase (Hudson 1994), much of this represented increases in NHS spending rather than spending on Local Authority social services.

Ironically, one of the other central acts of the Thatcher Government in the financing of services, and specifically of community care, was to have a crucial part to play in the array of forces that led to the major changes of the NHS and Community Care Act. This concerned changes in the regulations regarding payment of social security monies to provide an alternative to the fees paid by the Local Authority for residential care. In the spirit of the 'quasi-market' the Government sought to stimulate the growth of the so-called 'independent sector' by freeing up the limits on how much could be paid from social security monies for the fees of people in independent residential services. This resulted in a mushrooming of private and voluntary residential homes as a 'good investment' for financial entrepreneurs. It also, primarily in services for elderly people, enabled NHS managers to divest beds or close outright 'chronic care' hospitals and move people to independent nursing homes, thus diverting finance to the increased demands of the growth in 'high-tech' acute medicine. The side-effect of this, which the Government had clearly not foreseen, was a similar mushrooming of the social security budget. Despite benefits being cut in many other areas there was, between 1979 and 1989, a tenfold increase in this budget, from ten million to one hundred million pounds (Hudson 1994) and so, well before 1989, ministers were debating ways to maintain their Government's reputation as a cutter of public spending whilst at the same time keeping their support for the growing private care sector.

The community care solution – build up to the NHS and Community Care Act

If anything, the 'community care' strategy of the 1970s' Labour Government's strategy had been based on encouraging and facilitating change via existing organisational systems, with Health and Local Authorities continuing to have overlapping responsibilities. This relied on co-operation at the local level to move in the centrally desired directions. The Thatcher Government at first continued this policy, but became aware, as did others (Malin 1994) that the advocated switch from institutional to more local services was lagging well behind such targets as there were. In 1986, in *Making a Reality of Community Care*, the Audit Commission reviewed progress and analysed what it saw as the general failure of government implementation mechanisms. With these criticisms continuing, Mrs Thatcher turned to her trusted adviser from the business world, Sir Roy Griffiths, to find her an 'efficient' solution to the community care problem. His review, and the White Paper which followed, set a path towards the major organisational changes that were to emerge from the NHS and Community Care Act.

The review, published as the Griffiths Report (DoH 1988), was established to investigate the way in which public funds were being used to support community care policy and to advise on options for better use of those funds.

Its main recommendations were:

- Local Authority Social Service Departments should be responsible for identifying people with community care needs in their area and for negotiating with other authorities the contribution they would make to an individual's care and support needs.
- Assessment and Care Management, and the purchasing and provision of services to maintain or establish people in their own homes who might otherwise need to have institutional care, should be new powers added to Local Authority Social Services.
- An interactive planning relationship between Social Service Authorities, Health Authorities and other service-providing agencies was required.
- A Minister of State within the Department of Health should take responsibility for community care.

Government reaction to Griffiths came in a White Paper in 1989. It accepted key Griffiths recommendations but did not take on others, and its proposals may be seen as reflecting a fascinating amalgam of the 'new right' political philosophy discussed above, some practical organisational rearrangements, and some of the recommendations which had emerged over the previous twenty years regarding what constituted good quality local care.

The 1989 White Paper therefore set out six key objectives for service delivery:

- To promote the development of domiciliary, day and respite services to enable people to live in their own homes wherever feasible and sensible.
- To ensure that service providers make practical support for carers a high priority.
- To make proper assessment of need and good case management the cornerstone of high-quality care.
- To promote the development of a flourishing independent sector alongside good quality public services.
- To clarify the responsibilities of agencies and still make it easier to hold them to account for their performance.
- To secure better value for taxpayers' money by introducing a new funding structure for social care.

In then taking these objectives into legislation, however, the organisational and financial elements came to the fore. Possibly the recommendation from Griffiths that the Government had had most political difficulty in accepting was the proposal to hand over central responsibility for community care services to Local Authorities. This, as we have seen, ran counter to a general objective of the Thatcher Government to emasculate local government. The way the Government incorporated Griffiths' suggestion into their policy, however, still largely fitted that underlying objective. Responsibility was given to Local Authorities, but the legislation and direction ensured that the Local Authorities' role developed more as an 'enabler' – assessing need and arranging the purchase of care, mostly from elsewhere. The legislation also introduced major changes to the health services at the same time, thereby ensuring that the overall political imperative of a health and welfare market was created.

The NHS and Community Care Act 1990 – more NHS than community care

A major, but erroneous, public impression of the main impact of the NHS and Community Care Act was that it began the closure of hospitals and the onset of 'community care'. In fact, as we have seen, movement out of hospitals and ideas of community living had been going strong since the 1970s, led by the radical movements in learning disability and the practice of 'sheltered housing' for elderly people. In reality therefore, the vast bulk of the NHS and Community Care Act deals with major changes in the NHS, rather than community care. A simple examination of the contents reveals that, out of fifty-eight sections, forty-one have to do with changes to the NHS: the setting up of NHS Trusts and GP fund-holding practices; the various roles of commissioning and regulatory bodies; financial arrangements for transfer, etc. Even the community care sections are duplicated in terms of arrangements for England and Wales being followed by essentially the same provision for Scotland (nine and eight sections of the Act respectively).

Specifically the NHS and Community Care Act obliged Local Authorities to:

- produce Community Care Plans consistent with those of District Health Authorities (Section 46);
- develop an integrated system for assessing need, and the development of a system for designing packages of care and linking the delivery of services with resource allocations (Section 47); and
- establish 'arms length' units for inspection of residential services and units to receive and deal with complaints in respect of social care services (Section 48).

The rest of the 'community care' parts of the Act deal with more administrative detail on such things as transfers of finance and staff if services move from the NHS, but essentially the three sections above represent the main impact on Local Authorities.

The Department of Health then issued guidance on these and other areas of the Act, but left considerable scope for local decisions on the various systems to be used. In particular, advice was given on: assessment; care management; the introduction of a purchasing and contracting role as separate from the provision of services; and Local Authorities taking on responsibility for purchasing care in private and voluntary homes (DoHSSI 1991; DoH 1992).

What was all this to mean for the organisation and financing of services for people with learning difficulties? For those being served by the NHS, mostly those still in hospitals, though also a significant number in 'community projects', the immediate result was that their organisations joined the 'independent sector', as it came to be called. As we have seen, local political power in the NHS was not in the hands of elected politicians, and the NHS and Community Care Act had confirmed the arrangements, already started by a number of eager organisations, whereby the *provision* of health services was put in the hands of trusts, independently managed and governed. This effectively put them in a similar position to private and voluntary providers of health care, though the Government was keen to play down their effective privatisation by calling them 'NHS Trusts'.

Power over *expenditure* on learning disability services in the NHS, like all other *purchasing* decisions, was in the hands of the still centrally controlled (though renamed) NHS Executive, through District Health Authorities. Learning disability services would tend to be classified organisationally, at District Health Authority level, with other community care services. Again, therefore, the situation arose where managers in the new purchasing roles would have little knowledge of learning disability, and would be spending most of their time trying to empty the large hospitals, often with the trusts providing the 'community' alternative. Many learning disability trusts then sought to create a 'niche market' for themselves, especially in the area of so-called 'challenging behaviour'. Since the health authorities did not often have the expertise, but did have the finance, and also 'friends at court' in the shape of ex-NHS colleagues now in trusts, it is not surprising that the very variable quality found by Professor Mansell's team shortly afterwards was to emerge (Mansell 1993).

In Local Authorities, on the other hand, the 'purchaser/provider split', as it became regularly called, was much less uniformly implemented. Some authorities, believing in, or merely hoping for, a Labour victory in the 1992 election, did very little in the three-year implementation phase of the NHS and Community Care Act beyond what was absolutely mandated. Others, usually Conservative controlled authorities, made major changes very quickly, installing whole new sections to control purchasing and contracting, sometimes even physically separating them from the rest of the Social Services Departments. Lewis and Glennerster, who along with Wistow and his colleagues made major studies of the organisational impact of community care, found two, three or even four significant reorganisations in the authorities they studied, all within five years of the Act. They explain some of the reasons for this as follows:

It is very important to remember that the White Paper and Act do not specify in great detail how authorities must do things. Some requirements are very clear, such as that to set up an arms length inspection and complaints unit. Some are clear in that they must happen, but less prescriptive in how they are to be done. Assessment and care management is a good example of this. While the Department of Health and Social Services Inspectorate have offered many trees worth of advice, they have not required that a certain model be introduced. This is why we find very different implementation of the requirements in different authorities.

(Lewis and Glennerster 1996: 131)

Wistow *et al.*, who began their studies after the White Paper, are more direct in their analysis of the degree of change that the reforms would bring.

The development of such a purchasing function implied major changes in the organisation of departments which had traditionally had an administrative rather than a management culture. Indeed they required a strengthening of precisely those activities which had hitherto been most seriously under-developed in the planning and management of social service departments; the identification of needs, service design, service application and performance review. Moreover, in advocating enabling as a purchasing role, the White Paper was requiring departments to take on responsibilities for which they were ill equipped while simultaneously divesting themselves, at least in part, of the provider role which had traditionally been their area of relative management strength. Behind the apparent continuity suggested by the enabling terminology, therefore, lay a major break with previous policies for the personal social services. Although compulsory competitive tendering was explicitly rejected in the White Paper, its underlying objective was similar.

(Wistow *et al.* 1994: 16)

With the degree of organisational change that these authors and others found, the notion of 'managerialism' began to be promulgated as representing what was happening in the Social Services Departments, following its ready take up in the NHS. This has been defined in various ways (Cutler and Waine 1997) but the underlying theme is one of a belief that service agencies are no different to any other business organisation, delivering products to customers who need them, and therefore able to be managed by people who are good at management, rather than knowing about the particular product.

In exercises discussing this issue on the degree course at Stockport, students were given the task of looking at an organisation with which they were familiar, and discovering how it had changed since the NHS and Community Care Act. The most regular findings of these exercises fell into four main categories. First, those who knew about private or voluntary agencies remarked on the fact that they hadn't existed, or only in a small form, prior to the Act, but now were thriving. The second theme, regarding Health Trusts, initially differed from the rest of the independent sector, in that the trusts were running down as the hospitals closed, but later in the 1990s the results from the trusts began to fall in with the expansionary line of other private and voluntary agencies. Those who reported on Social Services Departments had much more mixed findings, reflecting in an anecdotal way the findings of Lewis and Glennerster (1996) about the much more patchy impact of managerialism, and attempts in a number of authorities to maintain 'professional' values and concerns, not least by continuing the requirement for managers to have professional qualifications.

All students, however, reported on a further phenomenon, which was the rapid rise of what one person called the 'suits, Filofaxes and mobile phones'. Put more soberly, the students reported almost unanimously of the change to services 'driven by money'. This, again, is an anecdotal reflection of the more formally organised research into the growth of managerialism. Though many found much to criticise in this movement (e.g. Hadley and Clough 1996), it is undoubtedly the case that, by the time of the 1997 election, the pattern of service organisation set up by and following the NHS and Community Care Act was so firmly ensconced that it was often difficult to discern any collective memory of things ever having been different.

For learning disability services the effects were perhaps felt more keenly than in other areas, because of the progress some services felt they had made in the 1970s and 1980s. As has been described elsewhere in this book, many service changes had come about as a result of the values-led 'movements' of that period, especially, as Emerson and Hatton (1996) note, as a result of normalisation. The big organisational changes, however, and the creation of the service marketplace meant that while some very good things could happen, mainly in the government favoured independent sector, some very bad things could also happen, given the lack of an overall strategy led by people who knew something about learning disability. As we have seen, learning disability services have always been near the bottom of the priority pile, but now, with the vast diffusion of different services from different sectors in any geographical area, Hadley and Clough's title, *Care in Chaos*, could certainly be said to apply in their case. 'Chaos', not just in the pejorative sense of disasters happening, but in the broader sense of no overall control or purpose. Perhaps things could 'only get better'.

The New Labour Government – modernising or controlling?

In trying to achieve a second term, four years after its landslide victory in May 1997, the New Labour Government made many claims regarding progress in what it chose to call its 'modernisation' agenda. Prominent among these were developments in health and social services, especially in terms of finance and organisational change, the subject of this chapter. Whether such changes have occurred, and whether they have resulted in improvements in services, needs to be set alongside, at least as far as learning disability services are concerned, the findings of the *Facing the Facts* national survey of 1999 (DoH 1999), and the need for further change identified in the White Paper *Valuing People* (DoH 2001).

In inheriting the full-blown social care market, nurtured through eighteen years of Conservative governments, and administered by cash-starved and politically neutered Local Authorities, the New Labour Government may have been tempted, as it appears to have been in other areas, to let things run for a while whilst it dealt with more easily addressed problems. If judged in terms of policy initiatives, however, the forests of paper and arachnoid armies of websites that emerged in the first four years of the government would argue against accusations of inertia.

Two key areas have, I would argue, remained unchanged. One is the use of the centralised power drawn to Westminster by Margaret Thatcher, though it has been used to impose the modernising agenda on the human service system, rather than to release still further the more rampant carnage of market forces. Nevertheless, the other area to remain has been the welfare market, despite some utterances to the contrary. It has remained, however, in a way which sought to level the playing field between public and private sector providers. In addition, as we shall see, though the idea of two separate functions of purchasing and providing have also remained, the developing policy advice and legislation has tended to push the two functions somewhat closer together organisationally. Much of this remains to be played out in practice however, so all this final section will attempt to do is to outline the intentions of policy and legislation relevant to the organisation and financing of learning disability services and look at some signs of what this might mean for the future.

Since the change of government the pace of change in public services has increased dramatically, not least in Social Services Departments and their partner agencies. Most of the changes are aimed, at least in the Government's rhetoric: at being better at working together – 'smarter working'; at being better at knowing how well services are doing – 'performance monitoring'; and at being better at using resources effectively – 'best value and efficiency'. Most have addressed issues at the macro level of the service organisations. As with events in the 1980s and 1990s, these changes have affected learning disability services as part of the wider picture, and they provide a framework of changes into which the more specific recommendations of the *Valuing People* White Paper can be fitted.

The most immediate came in the use of another of Thatcher's creations, at least in its revised role, the Audit Commission. Their report *The Coming of Age: Improving Care Services for Older People* (1997) points out key pressures on Community Care services for older people, repeating some of the criticisms of earlier in the decade concerning a vicious circle of antagonism between health and social services, and a blight on effective strategic planning. A government circular (*EL(97)62, Better Services for Vulnerable People*, DoH 1997) followed, and required Local Authorities and Health Authorities to work together to: agree a local Joint Investment Plan (JIP) for continuing and community care services for vulnerable people; improve the multi-disciplinary assessment process; and develop recuperation and rehabilitation services for older people. Government pressure continued in the Green Paper *Partnership in Action* (DoH 1998a), which set out proposals to improve joint working between Health and Social Services. It reinforced the idea of JIPs for a wider range of services and introduced the idea of Health Improvement Programmes (HImPs) as local strategies for improving healthcare linked to national targets. Many of these ideas were then included in later White Papers and legislation, including the key documents *Modernising Local Government*, (DETR 1998), which led to the Local Government Act of 1999; *The New NHS: Modern Dependable* (DoH 1998b), which led to the 1999 Health Services Act; and *Modernising Social Services* (DoH 1998c). Once again the key themes have many issues affecting learning disability services.

Modernising Local Government and the Local Government Act

The White Paper, and the legislation which followed, was an attempt by the Government to rescue the somewhat tarnished image of Local Authorities, but in such a way as to present the policy as not returning to the 'old Town Hall bureaucracy'. Key features included: the requirement to 'consider' replacement of the existing committee structure by an elected mayor or cabinet style government; a duty to consult local people on plans and services; and the idea of 'Beacon Councils' being rewarded for providing excellent performance as a target for others to aim at. This was sweetened by the abolition of universal council tax capping and the setting of the Standard Spending Assessment over three years to allow longer-term planning. To achieve results, however, the notion of 'Best Value' was to be introduced for all services. This again was taking the germ of a Thatcherite idea, 'value for money', but giving it a 'modern' spin by requiring authorities to subject their services to a process that became known as the 'four Cs' of 'Best Value'. These were as follows – for any Local Authority service, regardless of who provided it, there should be:

- *Challenge* – a questioning of why and how the service is being provided;
- *Comparison* – looking at that service in comparison with the performance of others;
- *Consultation* – with local taxpayers, service users and the wider business community on how that service could be improved; and
- *Competition* – fair competition, including the authority's own provided service, 'as a means to fair and effective services'.

Finally, to emphasise one of the key themes again, local performance plans were to be published and compared, leading to the first 'Corporate Performance Plans' league table in March 2000.

Social Services Departments were, of course, part of Local Authorities, and thus subject to the requirements of the Act. At the same time, however, they had to deal with their own White Paper.

Modernising Social Services

Published in November 1998, its subtitle *Promoting Independence; Improving Protection; Raising Standards* gives the clue to the thrust of policy. It argues that Social Services are supposed to be for the whole population, but have often failed to deliver required standards with respect to:

- protection of vulnerable individuals;
- co-ordination of different services;
- flexible responses to need;
- clarity of responsibility and role;
- consistency of response; and
- efficiency of service.

This amounted to quite a criticism of thirty years of Social Services Departments, and the White Paper implicitly criticises previous Labour administrations in rejecting a return to the 'Municipal Approach' to delivering large-scale public services. It is equally dismissive, however, of wholescale privatisation. Having criticised past performance, it then sets out principles for development of services, namely that services should:

- promote independence;
- meet individual needs;
- be delivered with fairness and consistency;
- provide a decent looked-after system;
- safeguard vulnerable people from abuse;
- have appropriately trained staff – to be facilitated by a new 'Social Care Council' with which staff must be registered; and
- have clear standards – including a Commission for Care Standards and a Social Care Institute of Excellence to parallel the National Institute of Clinical Excellence in the NHS.

Also of relevance here are the various grants to improve specific services, most of which require some form of partnership plan, especially the 'Partnership Grant' itself, which can only be awarded for plans agreed by all relevant authorities. This was designed to fit in with the third key White Paper and subsequent Act, that relating to the Health Service.

The New NHS: Modern Dependable and the 1999 Health Services Act

The White Paper and subsequent Act were seen as a prime example of a 'third way' approach to running the NHS, 'based on partnerships and driven by performance'. The link with the underlying themes should again be clear.

Key features were:

- The Health Improvement Programme – as described in *Partnership in Action* (DoH 1998a). These were to be introduced by April 2000.
- Primary Care Groups – the local organisation of the commissioning of 'primary care' including GPs – these were later to be developed into 'Primary Care Trusts' which combined the commissioning function with direct provision.
- A new statutory duty to work in partnership – this was then backed up with what became known as 'Health Act flexibilities', the ability of a partnership to use money that would have been ring-fenced for one activity in other activities in pursuit of the partnership objectives.
- Clinical Governance – a concept to try and ensure quality in all activities, using the notion of 'evidence-based practice' as its guide.
- The National Institute for Clinical Excellence (NICE) to be set up as a body to advise on clinical treatment and cost effectiveness.
- The ending of the 'internal market' in the NHS – this did not bring the trusts back into the NHS, they were to remain independent, but it did attempt to plan, through the primary care groups, local health services based on the sharing of information rather than the competitive secrecy that had been a feature of the early 1990s.

Organisational arrangements and *Valuing People*

As has been noted a number of times in this chapter, changes in the organisational arrangements and financing of learning disability services have always only been a part of wider changes in the service system. This has continued even in the strategy laid out in *Valuing People* despite its being purportedly specific to learning disability. In chapter 9 of that document, the organisational arrangements for the implementation of the strategy, known as Local Partnership Boards, are described as part of the 'overall framework provided by Local Strategic Partnerships' set up in the renewal/regeneration process described above for local agencies, including health and social services. As such they will be responsible, among other things, for the production of Joint Investment Plans, use 'Health Act flexibilities', and oversee local agency planning. The White Paper makes it clear that, while the chief executive of the local council is responsible for ensuring the Partnership Board is in place, the Boards 'will not be statutory bodies' and that, as well as representatives from social services, health authorities and primary care trusts, many other service agencies – education, housing, community development, leisure, the employment services and independent providers – are to be represented. So too, as full members, are representatives of carers and people with learning difficulties, including an emphasis on minority ethnic representation. The formation of these Boards is clearly a priority, with a deadline of October 2001, only some six months after the White Paper. Note, too, that the Boards are for adult services only, with services to children being part of generic Childrens' Services Plans.

What, then, might this mean for the development of services. At the start of this chapter, the idea of a unified service, common in the 1970s, was recalled. Attempts to get people involved in learning disability services to work together have been made ever since, though this chapter has argued that the wider events surrounding the NHS and Community Care Act have tended to fragment services, rather than bring them together. This seems to have been the result of both the purchaser/provider split and the emergence of the welfare market. Will the new Partnership Boards with the mandate to oversee 'the inter-agency planning and commissioning of comprehensive, integrated and inclusive services' be able to pull off the trick that has defeated even the best intentioned groups for thirty years or more? One suspects that the answer to that will lie, as it has before, in how much power and influence, and especially money, the dominant model of service, i.e the medical model in the broad sense of that word, is prepared to give up. Since no major organisational changes are suggested by the White Paper (though they do threaten to use powers under the Health and Social Care Act to impose arrangements if they are not put in place, including the possibility of 'Adult Trusts' to take over the commissioning function of Local Authorities), the real changes are coming in the planning and commissioning of services, rather than in their provision, and in the involvement, not just of the 'usual suspects' of health and social services, but service users and carers, and a host of other generic agencies. Pressure is also brought to bear in terms of the 'Health Act flexibilities', with funding for new developments only really being available from this source, which is itself dependent on organisations working together. Whether Boards will be able to use their power remains to be seen, and the presence of service providers on them lends a strange dynamic of self-interest, both from them and from the only other likely group who know about learning disabilities, the users and carers.

The Partnership Boards are also given the task of reviewing 'professional structures' especially learning disability teams, but also ensuring that 'organisational structures encourage and promote inclusive working with staff from the fields of housing, education, primary care, employment and leisure'. Though guidance is promised on the role of community teams, none is forthcoming on the form that these other organisational structures might take.

One is therefore left, as one's more naive self was twenty-five years ago, to ponder on the likelihood of organisations with different histories, different assumptions, vastly different knowledge of learning disability, and vastly different power positions both in terms of financial and professional power, coming together to form a seamless robe of service planning, still more implementation. Having said that, however, it appears to this rather less naive author that the White Paper represents the best chance in those twenty-five years of something positive happening, but with local leadership, whether in formal positions or otherwise, being the key to seizing that chance.

References

Acts of Parliament

National Health Service and Community Care Act (1990), London, HMSO.
Health Services Act (1999), London, The Stationery Office.
Local Government Act (1999), London, The Stationery Office.

General references

Audit Commission (1986) *Making a Reality of Community Care*, London, HMSO.
Audit Commission (1997) *The Coming of Age: Improving Care Services for Older People*, London, The Stationery Office.
Blunden, R. (1975) *The Development and Evaluation of Services for the Mentally Handicapped – An Outline Research Plan, Discussion Paper No. 2*. Mental Handicap in Wales – Applied Research Unit, Welsh National School of Medicine, Cardiff.
Cutler, T. and Waine, B. (1997) *Managing the Welfare State*, Oxford, Berg.
Department of the Environment, Transport and the Regions (1998) *Modernising Local Government*, London, The Stationery Office.
Department of Health (1988) *Community Care: Agenda for Action (The Griffiths Report)*, London, HMSO.
Department of Health (1989) *Caring for People: Community Care in the Next Decade and Beyond*, London, HMSO.
Department of Health (1992) *Memorandum on the Financing of Community Care Arrangements after April 1993 and on Individual Choice of Residential Accommodation*, London, Department of Health.
Department of Health (1997) *Circular EL (97)62, Better Services for Vulnerable People*, London, Department of Health.
Department of Health (1998a) *Partnership in Action, (New Opportunities for Joint Working between Health and Social Services), A Discussion Document*, London, The Stationery Office.
Department of Health (1998b) *The New NHS: Modern Dependable*, London, The Stationery Office.
Department of Health (1998c) *Modernising Social Services: Promoting Independence; Improving Protection; Raising Standards*, London, The Stationery Office.
Department of Health (1999) *Facing the Facts, Services for People with Learning Disabilities: A Policy Impact Study of Social Care and Health Services*, London, The Stationery Office.
Department of Health (2001) *Valuing People – a New Strategy for Learning Disability for the 21st Century*, London, The Stationery Office.
Department of Health and Social Security (1971) *Better Services for the Mentally Handicapped*, Command 4683, London, HMSO.
Department of Health Social Service Inspectorate (1991) *Care Management and Assessment: Summary of Practice Guidance*, London, HMSO.
Elliot J. (1975) Segregated ghetto or better services?, *Res. Soc. Work.*, 15, 4–5.
Emerson, E. and Hatton, C. (1996) *Residential Provision for People with Learning Disabilities: A Research Review*, Manchester, Hester Adrian Research Centre.

Hadley, R. and Clough, R. (1996) *Care in Chaos: Frustration and challenge in community care*, London, Cassell.

Home Office, Department of Education and Science, Ministry of Housing and Local Government, Ministry of Health (1968) *Report of the Committee on Local Authority and Allied Personal Social Services (The Seebohm Report)*, Command 3703, London, HMSO.

Hudson, R. (1994) Management and finance. In: N. Malin (ed.) *Implementing Community Care*, Buckingham, OUP.

Hutton, W. (1996) *The State We're In* (revised edition), London, Vintage Books.

Le Grand, J. (1990) *Quasi-Markets and Social Policy*, Bristol, School of Urban Studies, Bristol University.

Lewis, J. and Glennerster, H. (1996) *Implementing the New Community Care*, Buckingham, Open University Press.

Malin, N. (1994) Development of community care. In: N. Malin (ed.) *Implementing Community Care*, Buckingham, Open University Press.

Mansell, J. (1993) *Services for People with Learning Disabilities and Challenging Behaviour or Mental Health Needs, (The Mansell Report)*, London, HMSO.

Race, D.G. (1977) Investigation into the effects of different caring environments on the social competence of mentally handicapped adults, Unpublished PhD thesis – University of Reading.

Rowbottom, R. (1973) *Hospital Organisation*, London, Heinemann.

Rowbottom, R. (1974) *Social Services Department – Developing Patterns of Work and Organisation*, London, Heinemann Educational.

Shapiro, A. (1974) Fact and fiction in the care of the mentally handicapped, *Brit. J. Psychiat.*, 125: 286–92.

Thomas, D. (1973) A new caring profession – is it necessary? *Nursing Times*, 26 July.

Tizard, J. (1974) Services and the evaluation of services. In: A.M. Clarke and A.D.B. Clarke (eds) *Mental Deficiency – The Changing Outlook, 3rd edition*, London, Methuen.

Wistow, G., Knapp, M., Hardy, B. and Allen, C. (1994) *Social Care in Mixed Economy*, Buckingham, Open University Press.

Chapter 7

Evaluation of quality in learning disability services

Errol Cocks

Introduction

Quality is elusive in human services – hard to achieve and even harder to sustain. Quality can also be illusory, with much of the reality of the lives of vulnerable service users obscured by the rhetoric and technology of modern formal human services. The pursuit of quality has many purposes, some of them system-serving and some of them more human-focused. Modern formal human services have many characteristics, possibly the most challenging of which is that they serve multiple interests. Within this mass of vested interests, the most vulnerable people are usually the service users and there is a constant struggle to ensure that their interests are given priority against the interests of more powerful groups and systems.

The purpose of this chapter is to examine four approaches to the evaluation of quality in human services:

1 Human service evaluation instruments.
2 The model coherency of human services.
3 Quality of life.
4 Cultural value as a yardstick for quality.

The aim in describing these approaches is to draw out and illustrate the issues. A critical perspective will address the question of how priority is given to the needs and interests of service users. This reflects the concept of 'person centredness', a key objective identified in the *Valuing People* White Paper (DoH 2001). Note that this chapter is about people who are to some extent dependent upon *formal* human services. It does not consider informal ways in which people may be supported.

Before considering the four approaches, two recent important reports on quality in learning disability services are described, followed by some general issues about quality that set a necessary context for the chapter.

Two important reports – facing some facts

In 1999 the Department of Health released a report that represented a 'score card' of success in learning disability policy implementation over the past three decades

(DoH 1999). The Report described a major study of twenty-one local authorities and their partner health authorities that used surveys, field visits to ten of the authorities, and an analysis of national statistics. The study cited nine DoH policy reports published since 1992 that were relevant to learning disability. There was no shortage of these! The policy directions of these publications were consistent with the promotion of citizenship, social inclusion, community living, and the involvement and influence of service users and carers. These directions were well established in the learning disability field in the UK and internationally through the development of normalisation in the early 1970s, the 'Ordinary Life' initiative in the UK in the early 1980s, and the 'Care in the Community' initiatives of the late 1980s and early 1990s (see Chapter 2).

Although the Report documented some notable achievements, the findings and conclusions illustrated many poor outcomes.

1   Two thirds of people with learning difficulties:
     (a) lived in congregate care;
     (b) attended large, congregate day centres.
2   Almost 60 per cent of people living with carers had no regular respite.
3   Accessibility and appropriateness of services, especially for people with complex needs, was adversely affected by lack of clear organisational roles, service fragmentation, poor take-up of joint commissioning, little agreement on quality standards, and lack of performance monitoring and review.
4   Specialist services were reported as 'adequate' by less than half the authorities.
5   Basic data on services and service users was 'often lacking' and DoH statistics were of limited usefulness.
6   Care planning often resulted in negative carer experiences.
7   There was great variation in service quality across localities.

The Report concluded:

> All of these authorities can demonstrate examples of significant improvements in practice. However, the overall conclusion reached from the detailed analysis of current services must be that the realisation of the 'better life' principles was a long way off for most service users.
>
> The process of transforming the more congregate forms of accommodation and care into more individualised support in one's home or other homely surroundings appears to have faltered during the last decade.
>
> (DoH 1999: 31)

An earlier report (Emerson *et al.* 1999) described a major UK study commissioned by the DoH to explore the nature, quality and costs of residential or village communities, and community-based dispersed housing schemes for people with learning disabilities. The study reviewed the UK literature since 1980s and gathered data on service settings, client characteristics, views of relatives, and service costs from a random sample of 500 service users in eighteen services. The study methodology controlled for ability and challenging behaviour, variables known to influence service outcomes. This enabled 'like by like' comparisons to be made. The key findings provided a further reflection of quality issues in UK learning disability services.

Poor quality was found across *all forms* of service provision. This is consistent with a substantial volume of UK and international research. Being small and community-based are not sufficient conditions for quality. However, residential campuses arising from hospital contractions or closures were of significantly poorer quality than dispersed housing on a wide range of measures of benefits. The researchers stated: 'the process of hospital closure should be completed by the re-provision of the remaining hospital-based services within small community-based dispersed housing schemes' (Emerson *et al.* 1999: 18) The cost differential between campus and community re-provision was £6,000 (12 per cent) in favour of campus re-provision; however, any account of the *cost–benefit* of different service models should include a wide range of substantial client benefits that accompanied the dispersed service model. The researchers recommended that Local Authorities commission campus re-provision in terms of *both* the needs and wishes of service users and carers, *and* cost–benefit. It was recommended that supported living schemes should be included in permissible options.

The Report recommended that a more comprehensive range of quality indicators be developed and applied routinely. Broad indicators such as the number of people in a residence or service costs were inadequate measures of quality and outcome.

These reports are the most recent attempts to evaluate the state of services for people with learning difficulties in the UK. They illustrate that in spite of years of well-grounded policy development, implementation is patchy and quality is wanting. It is notable that the *Facing the Facts* report provided a stimulus for the initiation of the White Paper (DoH 2001) and the recommendations of Emerson *et al.* are largely taken up by that document.

Some general issues of quality in formal human services

A simple systems model

From time to time in this chapter I will refer to a simple systems model of human services that helps to frame the issues. This model has three elements.

1   *Inputs*: the resources that go into human services, e.g., human, financial and physical resources.
2   *Processes*: the ways in which a service uses the inputs, e.g., what a service does to, or for, service users, and how it does it.

3   *Products*: these consist of *outputs* such as the number of places provided in a service, and *outcomes* such as the impact of the service on service users.

Quality initiatives will usually focus on one or more of these elements.

Different perspectives on quality

A small Australian study from the 1970s explored the meaning of 'independence' for adults with learning disabilities, their parents, and support workers. Although there was agreement, there were significant differences between the three groups. For example, the service users viewed independence as having their own place in which to live. Parents viewed independence as their sons or daughters being able to keep their homes clean and being safe. Service providers, suitably imbued with ideological fervour, saw independence in terms of the people making their own decisions. Views of quality will reflect the needs and interests of each stakeholder group. One's ideological position may dictate that one group or another should always have priority, but the situation is more complex than that. Although the service providers' perspectives were valid and defensible, they needed to be leavened by issues of capacity and risk, and also take into account the importance of their families to the service users. These are difficult differences to resolve and they require careful consideration and good communication between the various parties.

Establishing criteria for quality

Assumptions and values

The criteria used to conceptualise and measure quality in human services must be based on assumptions and values that are consistent with the interests of service users. Sometimes, the criteria may rest upon faulty assumptions or poor values. In Australia in the early 1980s, a formal inquiry into a large institution in Melbourne essentially concluded that demonstrably poor services were appropriate for the service users because they were perceived to have insufficient potential to benefit from living in the community. This powerful assumption unfortunately remains prevalent in services for people with disabilities, especially for people with complex needs such as the large number of people who are in 'continuing care' services on hospital sites in the UK. When the Victorian institution was eventually closed and the residents moved into small community homes, the inquiry's assumptions proved faulty.

Formality

Some services may have limited 'corporate' identity because they have little in the way of formal documentation, policies, records, etc.; however, they may provide services that are highly valued by service users. In contrast, coldly professionalised services may have plenty of formality and regulation, but may not address adequately the human needs of service users. Some approaches to evaluating service quality may penalise the first service and reward the second.

System needs

As human services have become larger and more formal, the needs of the 'system' have become increasingly dominant. System needs provide a powerful call on resources in human services. They are reflected in the burgeoning of policies, regulations and accountability requirements. Increasing time of human service workers is taken up with 'paperwork' requirements and other activities that seem remote from the reasons why many people came into human services as a career – to promote the interests of service users. System requirements have strongly influenced the way in which quality is viewed in human services.

Triviality

It is common in human service to find quality defined and measured in relatively trivial terms, particularly so because of ease of measurement. For example, measurement of the quality of individual programme plans, especially when mandated by legislation or regulation, may be confined to the number of plans completed. This is an *output* measure and does not take into account aspects such as the quality of the planning processes, the extent to which plans were implemented, and the *outcomes* for service users. The latter considerations are much more complex than a simple frequency measure.

Measuring the right thing

From the standpoint of service users' needs, service quality measures may address the wrong thing. Services that are primarily custodial or protective may see quality as the provision of a degree of basic physical care and security, but may overlook the vital developmental needs of service users. In residential services, a common *process* quality measure relates to the number of people sharing a bedroom. While relevant for some, for many people, sharing a bedroom with a partner is desirable. The key to measuring the 'right' thing is the close knowledge of service users and the way in which their needs are identified and prioritised.

Universality

There is a dilemma in applying universal standards of quality across many or all services of a particular type, and all service users. On the one hand, concern about poor quality may require the establishment of minimally acceptable standards. On the other hand, universal standards limit flexibility, cannot take individual needs into account, and are also likely to set goals that are too low.

The relationship between processes, outputs and outcomes

There is a complex relationship between processes, outputs and outcomes in considering quality.

- Quality defined as *output* is likely to overlook the perspectives of key stakeholders including service users and carers. Consideration of the *outcomes* of a service are more likely to address how a service impacts on these groups.
- Although all approaches to conceptualising quality rest upon assumptions and values, a focus on outcomes is more likely to require a theoretical framework such as normalisation, social integration, empowerment, etc.
- Processes in human services are a vital aspect of quality. Measurement of outputs or outcomes does not necessarily reveal *how* they were achieved and this will have a fundamental influence on quality, especially from the perspective of service users. A service that successfully reduces the challenging behaviour of a service user may achieve this by using harmful processes. Perhaps medication has dire side-effects, the service user's rights are abrogated, or the processes are punitive. The service user may be institutionalised with eight other people who present similar behaviours. Because modern formal human services are so focused on getting certain results, there may be insufficient attention given to the price paid by the service user through the use of harmful processes.
- In human services, outcomes may be processes. The decision about at which point to measure quality may be somewhat arbitrary. Quality may be defined as the achievement of a job, or relocation into a small community house. However, the job may involve dangerous or demeaning work or low recompense. Because of lack of other supports, community living may mean social isolation. It may be more relevant to think of a job or a place to live as a *means* or process by which outcomes of financial independence or personal development are achieved. A useful reflection here is how the relocation of disabled people into 'the community' may be driven by person-centred agendas rather than agendas concerned with the number of people moved, reduction in institutional places, or alternative uses for institutional sites.

These issues emphasise the importance of clarity about the assumptions and values that underpin consideration of quality.

Human service evaluation instruments

Many instruments have been designed specifically to measure aspects of quality in human services. We will examine two approaches. The first considers two instruments, PASS and PASSING (Wolfensberger and Glenn 1973, Wolfensberger and Thomas 1983), designed to measure the extent to which a service achieves outcomes based on normalisation and Social Role Valorisation (SRV) (see also Chapter 11). The second describes the use of multiple measures of quality. We begin with five important preliminary considerations.

Human service evaluation instruments have different purposes

- *Evaluation* of some aspect/s of service quality, which itself may have a purpose, e.g., meeting funding requirements.
- *Research*, particularly to make comparisons between different service models, or the same service at different points in time.
- *Service development*, involving the use of the evaluation tool to advise on service changes.
- *Training* for human service workers and other stakeholders, e.g., training evaluations, using the tool to teach about aspects of human services.

Evaluation instruments are usually focused on processes and outcomes

Evaluation tools are often concerned with *how* a service operates and with outcomes for service users. They may incorporate output type measures, but more often they are concerned with impact on service users.

Evaluation instruments may focus on particular types of services or service user groups

For example, PASS and PASSING apply to all types of human services and service user groups. The second approach describes multiple measures that are confined to residential services for adults with learning difficulties.

Evaluation instruments may have been developed from particular conceptual or theoretical perspectives

PASS is based on normalisation, and PASSING on Social Role Valorisation. Some multiple measures have clear conceptual or theoretical links, for example, measures related to social integration or choice, and others do not. Multiple measures may have other pragmatic rationales. The evaluator may design the combination of measures according to the particular demands of the situation. Where multiple measures are used in a research context, the measures chosen may reflect the nature of the research questions being asked, or may be following a line of inquiry established over a period of time.

The statistical properties of evaluation instruments are important

All these purposes require that an evaluation instrument has certain characteristics, many of which relate to properties that can be statistically determined. These include:

- An acceptable level of *reliability* of measurement, i.e., the instrument has sufficient standardisation so that consistent results will be obtained over time and if more than one person uses the instrument in an evaluation process.
- An acceptable level of *validity*, i.e., it can be shown that the instrument is measuring what it is intended to measure.
- Sufficient *user friendliness*, i.e., the instrument is practically usable.

When choosing an evaluation instrument, an evaluator will pay close attention to these characteristics and may take reliability measures routinely during the evaluation.

PASS and PASSING

These instruments are derived from conceptual and theoretical schemas. They were designed to address all of the above purposes: evaluation, research, service development, and training. Although they developed in the context of learning disability services, they can be used to evaluate all forms of human services for any service user group. Because the instruments are based on explicit conceptual and theoretical foundations (i.e., normalisation and SRV), they are of limited use if the purposes of the evaluation are not consistent with those foundations. Both instruments measure aspects of a service against an *optimal standard* and use a quantitative approach. Because of this rigour, services commonly achieve relatively low scores, which tests the resolve of the service and the evaluators! In contrast, many evaluation instruments adopt a minimal or average standard, or simply make comparisons between services without recourse to an ideal standard or benchmark. PASS and PASSING have been used in the USA, Canada, the UK, Australia, New Zealand, Scandinavia and France. There is a database of many hundreds of PASS and PASSING evaluations and we will consider below some of the conclusions drawn from that data. This description is largely confined to PASSING.

The structure of PASS and PASSING

Program Analysis of Service Systems (PASS) (Wolfensberger and Glenn, 1973) is a fifty-item scale consisting of two sets of ratings. The first set measures administrative aspects of a service, based on some concepts developed in Nebraska and Canada in the late 1960s and early 1970s that are related to comprehensive service systems. The second set of ratings measures aspects of a service according to normalisation principles.

Program Analysis of Service Systems' Implementation of Normalisation Goals (PASSING) (Wolfensberger and Thomas, 1983) has forty-two ratings, all of which are based on the more recent development of SRV theory. The structure of PASSING closely reflects the theory and it is instructive to examine how this is so.

As discussed in Chapter 11, SRV theory (Wolfensberger, 1983a, 2000) is concerned with *social devaluation*, the according of low social value to certain individuals and groups in society. This makes the theory especially relevant to human services because many clients of human services experience, or are vulnerable to, social devaluation. SRV examines how social devaluation occurs and how it impacts on people and society, and describes strategies to counter it. The theory can be outlined concisely as follows:

1   A key goal suggested by SRV in addressing social devaluation is to promote the *valued social roles* of people who are at risk of social devaluation. This occurs through enabling vulnerable people to maintain valued roles such as family member, student, worker, citizen, and friend, and avoiding devalued roles such as menace, eternal child, sick person, object of pity, etc. (see Table 11.1).

2   The two key strategies suggested by SRV through which valued roles are achieved are:
    (a) to enhance a person's social image; and
    (b) to enhance a person's competencies.

3   Within human services, these strategies are achieved by working through a number of *media*, including:
    (a) physical settings of services;
    (b) relationships and groupings mediated by the service;
    (c) activities and time usage within the service; and
    (d) use of language and other symbols and images used by the service (see Table 11.2).

Table 7.1 illustrates the close link between structure and theory in PASSING.

Each of the forty-two PASSING ratings is scored on a five-point scale and is then accorded a particular *weight* that is based upon the relative importance of the rating in terms of SRV theory. For example, the rating concerned with the extent to which the service addresses the needs of service users has a higher weight than the rating that assesses the impact of the prior history of the service setting. In an evaluation, a service would have forty-two separate rating scores. These are combined in a number of ways, such as the total score, scores for image enhancement and competency enhancement, and scores for each of the seven categories listed in Table 7.1.

Evaluations using PASSING are meant to follow a relatively standardised process, which is spelled out in considerable detail (Wolfensberger 1983b). This manual is valuable in any form of human service evaluation, not only those based on normalisation or SRV.

Table 7.1 The structure of PASSING and its relationship to SRV theory

	1 Programme elements related primarily to social image enhancement	*2 Programme elements related primarily to competency enhancement*
01 Physical setting of service	11 ratings	6 ratings
02 Service-structured groupings and relationships among people	7 ratings	6 ratings
03 Service-structured activities and other uses of time	3 ratings	3 ratings
04 Miscellaneous other service language, symbols and images	6 ratings	No ratings – not applicable.

Source: Wolfensberger and Thomas 1983: 5.

PASS and PASSING conclusions on service quality

There is a substantial database of PASS and PASSING evaluations (Cocks 1998; Flynn 1999; Flynn *et al.* 1999). Some of the conclusions drawn from the data follow:

1 Overall, the quality of human service programmes when measured against the rigorous criteria of PASS and PASSING is 'modest' (Flynn 1999). In two large samples of evaluations, the average score on PASS (626 service evaluations) was 43 per cent of the possible total score, and on PASSING (633 service evaluations) it was 32 per cent. The difference between the two averages is largely accounted for by the inclusion in PASS of the administration ratings on which services tend to do better.

2 The instruments had sound statistical properties. For example, they discriminated between service types and service user groups. When particular service types were compared, vocational programmes, community-based programmes, and family and children's services achieved better scores than forms of institutional services.

3 In line with a growing volume of international research, PASS and PASSING evaluations showed that services achieved higher scores on *structural* features of services than on *functional* features. Structural features included where a service was located, its physical characteristics, the achievement of *physical* integration and community *presence*, etc. Functional features included the day-to-day operation of services, achievement of *social* integration and community *participation*, relationships, addressing developmental needs, etc.

4 Key service quality issues that remained particularly elusive included:

(a) understanding the needs of service users;

(b) the *relevance* and *effectiveness* of the service response to needs, developmental needs in particular; and

(c) the independence and social integration of service users.

Multiple measures

It is common for service evaluations to use a number of different measures to address different aspects of services. This approach is pragmatic, reflecting the focus of the particular evaluation and possibly drawing on a number of conceptual or theoretical elements. The study described briefly below illustrates this approach.

Felce *et al.* (2000) studied the relationship between quality and the costs of residential services for adults with severe learning disabilities and severe challenging behaviours in two service types – traditional services and new, specialised community housing. Altogether, the study used nineteen measures that related to five 'themes'.

1 Characteristics and behaviours of residents were described using schedules that assessed behavioural characteristics and adaptive behaviour.

2 Characteristics of the service settings were assessed including: the size, nature and location of the service; the characteristics of resident groups; staffing; adaptation of buildings; and staff working methods.

3 Service processes and resident outcomes were assessed using schedules and direct observation of staff–resident interactions.

4 Quality of life of service users was assessed with measures of community involvement, participation in the domestic life of the residence and the achievement of adult autonomy.

5 There were various measures of service costs.

The use of multiple measures of quality is often associated with research purposes and involves multivariate statistical analysis. In this case, Felce *et al.* (2000) concluded that there was a 'weak linear relationship between resource inputs and service quality'. Similarly, the relationship between resource inputs (costs) and quality of life was not straightforward. For example, larger numbers of staff were associated with *lower* resident autonomy. Previous research also has shown that larger numbers of staff are associated with *lower* levels of staff–resident interaction.

This study is one of a long tradition of using multiple quality measures in a research context (e.g., Hatton *et al.* 1995; Emerson *et al.* 1999).

The model coherency of human services

The model coherency concept

Model coherency originally was a rating in PASS and has been developed considerably since the early 1970s (Cocks 2001). It asks the most basic of questions related to service quality:

> Are the right people working with the right clients, who are properly grouped, doing the right thing, using the right methods, and consistently so?

The concept assumes that high human service quality is directly related to the extent of coherency between *what* a human service does, *how* it does it, and the *needs* of the service users.

An important related concept is that of *programmatic* and *non-programmatic* activities in human services. Programmatic activities are *directly related to addressing the needs of service users*. These include how needs are identified, physical aspects of a service, how a service groups the service users, and the methods used to support them. Non-programmatic activities include how a service addresses the needs of other stakeholders such as staff, funders, and organisations. Although non-programmatic activities may influence service quality, the *essence* of service quality is contained in programmatic activities. In fact many non-programmatic issues are not related directly to the needs of service users and may even not be in their best interests. It is an important reflection that as modern formal human services become more bureaucratic, rule-governed, and system-serving, some programmatic issues may be forced out. Model coherency is concerned with programmatic issues, not the non-programmatic.

Model coherency is also based on the assumption that all types of human services for all groups of service users share *universal characteristics*. However, modern formal human services are based more on a reductionist assumption that leads to high levels of specialisation between services and a decided lack of integrated, 'joined-up thinking'. Although reductionism and specialisation provide definite benefits, these characteristics create barriers that fragment the dissemination of knowledge across different human services and professions. Model coherency uses a universal framework that can be applied to all types of human services for all types of service recipients. The framework, called a *human service model*, consists of four *elements*.

1   *The key assumptions about important, relevant aspects of a human service.* Every human service is based on assumptions about the *parameters* of the social or human problem being addressed. These include:
    (a) the nature of the problem;
    (b) the factors that contribute to it;
    (c) effective responses to it; and
    (d) desired outcomes from human services.

For example, services for people with learning difficulties are still powerfully influenced by the assumption that the problem is medical (biological) and these people, or at least many of them, are patients who require hospitalisation, etc.

2   *The people who are the intended beneficiaries or recipients of the service.* This is concerned with the *needs* of service users. How a service thinks about and identifies service users' needs is fundamental to the relevance and effectiveness of a service. Human services may provide what they have always provided or have the capacity to provide, rather than what service users *need.* In the application of model coherency, which will be discussed below, the concept of needs takes different forms. Some needs are universal in that *all* human beings have them, including people with profound disabilities. Some needs are specific and specialised, and relate to the characteristics of individuals. Needs differ according to the degree of *urgency* they have for individuals. Often, urgent needs, such as security and belonging, must be addressed before other needs can be.

3   *The service content/s, i.e., what the service is giving to the service recipients.* The content of a human service refers to *what* it is that a human service conveys to service users and is distinguished from *how* this is done (the service *processes*). Service content is related to the needs of service users. There are a relatively limited number of contents but a limitless number of processes by which those contents can be provided. Three of the most common service contents for disabled people are better health, competencies and security.

4   *The processes by which the service provides the service content/s.* A human service delivers its contents through processes incorporated into four categories.
    (a) methods and technologies, including both the physical characteristics of the service and the 'treatments' provided by the service;
    (b) the language used by the service, e.g., about the service users and methods used.
    (c) the various groupings of service users created by the service; and
    (d) the characteristics of the people who provide the service.
    Within these categories, there are many different processes.

The application of model coherency

Model coherency is used in a number of different ways, each of which addresses issues of service quality.

1   The framework of a human service model enables the *description* of a human service. A service evaluation can:
    (a) identify many of the influential assumptions that underpin the service;
    (b) consider who are the service users and describe their needs;
    (c) identify the service contents; and
    (d) describe the various processes used by the service.

2   Once described, it becomes possible to *analyse* and *evaluate* a service using the model framework. A key issue here is the extent to which the various elements of the model are *coherent*, that is, fit together. Examples of poor quality (incoherency) may come from:

   (a) incorrect assumptions about important matters such as the nature of the problem; and

   (b) mismatches between service users' needs and the content/s chosen by the service, and/or the processes used.

   For example, the assumption that people with learning difficulties are sick (and they are not) may lead to important developmental needs being overlooked, an unnecessary emphasis on physical health, and service users being hospitalised and cared for by medical personnel. A model coherency analysis would draw out the incoherency in such a service.

3   Model coherency can be used to design or plan a new service for an identified group of service users.

4   Model coherency can provide training opportunities for human service workers and other stakeholders. This might be done through a training analysis of a service or a planning exercise around a hypothetical group of service users.

Model coherency has great value in enabling people to gain insights into the way human services are structured and operate, and how these influence service quality. It remains a rare and important theoretical framework for the description and analysis of human service programmes. Note that the model coherency process focuses on groups of service users and does not lend itself easily to an individualised approach.

Quality of life

Concepts of quality of life (QoL)

There is a long tradition of using statistics, indices and indicators of various kinds to measure and make comparisons between aspects of the health and well-being of populations. For example, comparisons of the standard of living across different countries may be measured in part by the possession of consumer goods such as motor vehicles and refrigerators. The health of nations may be assessed by the proportion of government revenues allocated to health services, the proportion of children who are immunised against common diseases, or the number of GPs. Bodies such as the Organisation for Economic Cooperation and Development and the World Health Organization collect and disseminate comparative statistics that are often turned into 'league tables', sometimes to the embarrassment of countries that do not do so well. In the 1970s and 1980s, the notion of quality of life (QoL) began to be applied to human service contexts and now it constitutes a major focus of outcome evaluation research in services for people with learning difficulties.

QoL can be defined as an assessment of a person's perception of his/her life experiences and conditions. The assessment can be through self-report or from the perceptions of another person (called a *proxy*). These assessments are considered to be *subjective*. QoL also may be measured indirectly by assuming that a particular life condition (such as illness, institutionalisation, wealth, employment) will be related to a particular level of QoL. Such assessment may be considered to be *objective* in that the life conditions may be derived from scores on a service quality measure.

Measurement of quality of life

In evaluation exercises, QoL becomes *operationalised* into indicators. Referring back to the simple systems model with which we began, QoL can be thought of as an outcome and thus draws on conceptual or theoretical considerations. For example, one way of conceptualising QoL is illustrated by *Quality of life accomplishments* (O'Brien 1987) which were derived from normalisation. These five accomplishments, community presence, community participation, choice, competency and respect, represent dimensions of quality in a person's life and lend themselves to both measurement and action in human service contexts. There are many different QoL measurement instruments (Goode 1994).

Three important areas of living are often incorporated into QoL measures.

1   Home and community living, which might include some assessment of safety and security, and social interactions.
2   Engagement in meaningful activities, including paid work.
3   Health functioning such as mobility and physical health.

Some issues with quality of life

Issues with the concept and application of QoL illustrate dilemmas in formal human services.

1   QoL is a very subjective concept which presents many problems of definition and measurement. QoL is not a very stable concept, varying with the circumstances and feelings of a person from one time period to another.
2   There are discrepancies in the measurement of QoL between self-reported and proxy assessment of QoL, suggesting that it is difficult for one person to judge the QoL of another. Commonly, proxy measures are lower than self-reported QoL. Decisions made on the basis of proxy assessments of QoL may lack validity.
3   A related issue is that there is not a clear relationship between *objective* measures of QoL and self-reports. For example, evaluation of *service quality* may not correspond with how an individual feels about his/her life. People who have lived much of their lives in poor quality institutional settings may

report satisfaction with many aspects of life and may resist attempts to convince them otherwise. Limited life experiences may not allow people to realise what life could be like. A single aspect of a person's life, for example an important relationship, may influence that person's entire perception of life.

4   Both of the preceding issues make decision making on the basis of QoL very questionable indeed. A major criticism of QoL is that it is used to make life-defining decisions, even life and death decisions, about vulnerable people. QoL may be equated with *the value of a person's life* (Wolfensberger 1994).

Cultural value as a yardstick for quality

When Nirje (1969) first wrote about normalisation, in a somewhat poetic way, he described how people with 'mental retardation' should be enabled to experience 'the normal rhythms of life'. He was responding to the realities of the deprived lives of people who lived in large institutions in Scandinavia and elsewhere in the world. He incorporated notions of the normal rhythm of the day, the week, the year, and of life, and in doing so drew attention to the richness and variety of ordinary life experience that should be available for the people about whom he wrote. In spite of the confusions and controversies about what is 'normal' and what isn't, and the 'celebration of difference', these ideas remain important for human services.

Wolfensberger developed the notion of what is normal or ordinary into the concept of *cultural value*. Whereas the concept of normal implies some sort of statistical judgement, cultural value implies that something has a history of being useful, familiar, and desired. If applied to human services, this concept could provide a yardstick by which service quality could be evaluated. The rationale for this approach is that if a human service measure is perceived by people to be useful, familiar and desired, rather than being strange and possibly even to be feared, then the people who use that measure are likely to benefit from that perception. For example, providing a home in a valued residential neighbourhood rather than a large, isolated, institutional setting is likely to reflect better on both the residents and the service providers.

This concept can be operationalised by applying the yardstick of how well any service measure (e.g., providing a place to live) reflects the diversity of culturally valued alternatives according to the manner in which the corresponding need is met for ordinary citizens. To illustrate this, we can ask: 'What are the characteristics of a house that is *not* a home in the sense of cultural value?' It might have these characteristics:

1   Planned from a common human service 'formula' (e.g., a group home, hostel or nursing home) rather than planned specifically for the people who live there.

2   Run according to the requirements and needs of the service system, e.g., paid carers, unions, professionals, rosters, regulations, funding requirements,

occupational health and safety, intake and assessment systems, policies, standards, licensing, etc.

3   People living there have little or no input into the home practices or influence in who may live with them.

4   People move in and out, perhaps because the home provides 'respite' short stays.

5   Co-residents are chosen because they have perceived similar problematic characteristics such as 'challenging behaviour' or old age.

6   Little opportunity is provided for residents' individuality to be expressed.

And so on . . .

Applying the yardstick of cultural value, the quality of the home would be evaluated not against the extent to which it abided by regulations, but by the extent to which it reflected the culturally valued idealisation of home – perhaps even reflecting the homes of human service workers themselves! We might then describe common *home forming practices*.

The following list is drawn from the work of Michael Kendrick:

1   The location of the home is suited to the person's needs, tastes, and necessities.

2   Ownership or tenancy responsibilities are carried by the person or someone designated to act for the person.

3   Scrupulous attention is paid to the selection of persons, if any, with whom the home is shared.

4   Bureaucratic practices are minimised.

5   Staff, family and service agency 'idealise' the ethic of 'home'.

6   Staff respect the sanctity of home for the people who live there.

7   There is conscious creation of experiences that promote intimacy and sharing in the home, including a spirit of welcome, hospitality and sharing with non-residents.

8   Conditions are created that enable people to face sorrows, setbacks and hardships of life.

9   There is loving upkeep of the home and support to face the responsibilities and obligations of maintaining a home.

10   There is meticulous attention paid to the tastes, preferences and expressions of the resident about his/her home.

11   Staff with a 'calling' for home are recruited, selected, and fostered.

12   Where supervision is required, it is provided in a manner consistent with this being the person's home.

This is a challenging list of quality indicators for any human service to work on. One could apply a similar approach to developing indicators of service quality in vocational, employment and educational services, for example. Rather than following the familiar route in human service analysis and planning and do what other formal human services have done with the particular service user group, the yardstick would be what is culturally valued.

At the same time, formal human services can never become entirely what they are setting out to replace but can only work towards and approximate it. It is also the case that because of the particular risks of human services, some degree of formality cannot be avoided, although it can be sensibly minimised. The pendulum may swing too far towards the formalised, regulated end or too much towards the risky end where there are few formal safeguards in place. The heart of the matter is whether the people who plan and provide services retain the capacity to acknowledge that people who use human services share universal needs and are not the sum of their impairments.

Conclusions

This account of the pursuit of quality has taken a necessarily critical perspective on human services. This comes from mounting evidence that many human services are in crisis and some are inflicting harm on vulnerable people. This is a bitter pill to swallow for human service workers who are committed to the people they serve and only wish to do well by them. Nevertheless, a deeper understanding of what it is about human services and society that contributes to poor quality outcomes in human services is an essential first step to improvement. At the same time, a particularly critical perspective is required about the reliance on ever-increasing formality and technology as an antidote to the limitations of human services. In many respects, these contribute to the very dynamics that erode quality by squeezing the *human* out of human services.

At the outset, I stated that this chapter was about formal human services and not about informal ways of supporting and helping. Possibly it is in this range of societal responses that an alternative paradigm may emerge (or re-emerge). In this regard, the positive impact of vulnerable people having a strong voice, the influence of advocates and allies, and the alternative perspectives of aspects of the social model of disability provide hope. In the meantime, there remains much to do within formal human services upon which so many vulnerable people are dependent.

References

Cocks, E. (1998) Evaluating the quality of residential services for people with disabilities using Program Analysis of Service Systems' Implementation of Normalization Goals (PASSING), *Asia and Pacific Journal on Disability*, 1 (2): 29–41.

Cocks, E. (2001) Model coherency analysis and the evaluation of human service quality, unpublished manuscript, Western Australia, Curtin University of Technology.

Department of Health (1999) *Facing the Facts. Services for People with Learning Disabilities: A Policy Impact Study of Social Care and Health Services*, London, DoH.

Department of Health (2001). *Valuing People. A New Strategy for Learning Disability for the 21st Century*, London HMSO.

Emerson, E., Robertson, J., Gregory, N., Hatton, C., Kessissoglou, S., Hallam, A., Knapp, M., Jarbrink, K., Netten, A. and Walsh, P. (1999) *Quality and Costs of Residential Supports for People with Learning Disabilities: A Comparative Analysis of Quality and Costs in Village Communities, Residential Campuses and Dispersed Housing Schemes.* Manchester: Hester Adrian Research Centre, University of Manchester.

Felce, D., Lowe K., Beecham, J. and Hallam, A. (2000) Exploring the relationships between costs and quality of services for adults with severe intellectual disabilities and the most severe challenging behaviours in Wales: A multivariate regression analysis. *Journal of Intellectual & Developmental Disability*, 25 (4): 307–326.

Flynn, R.J. (1999) A comprehensive review of research conducted with the program evaluation instruments PASS and PASSING. In: R. J. Flynn and R. A. Lemay (eds) *A Quarter-century of Normalisation and Social Role Valorisation: Evolution and Impact,* Ottawa, Canada: University of Ottawa Press.

Flynn, R. J., Guirguis, M., Wolfensberger, W. and Cocks, E. (1999) Cross-validated factor structures and factor-based subscales for PASS and PASSING, *Mental Retardation*, 37 (4): 281–296.

Goode, D.A. (ed.) (1994) *Quality of Life for Persons with Disabilities: International Perspectives and Issues*, Cambridge, MA, Brookline Books.

Hatton, C., Emerson, E., Robertson, J., Henderson, D. and Cooper, J. (1995) The quality and costs of residential services for adults with multiple disabilities: A comparative evaluation, *Research in Developmental Disabilities*, 16 (6): 439–460.

Nirje, B. (1969) The Normalisation principle and its human management implications. In: R.B. Kugel and W. Wolfensberger (eds) *Changing Patterns in Residential Services for the Mentally Retarded*, Washington, DC, President's Committee on Mental Retardation.

O'Brien, J. (1987) A guide to lifestyle planning. In: B. Wilcox and T. Bellamy (eds) *A Comprehensive Guide to the Activities Catalogue*, Baltimore, MD, Paul Brookes Publishing Co.

Wolfensberger, W. (1983a) Social role valorization: A proposed new term for the principle of normalisation, *Mental Retardation*, 21 (6): 234–239.

Wolfensberger, W. (1983b) *Guidelines for Evaluators During a PASS, PASSING, or Similar Assessment of Human Service Quality*, Toronto, ONT, National Institute on Mental Retardation.

Wolfensberger, W. (1994). Let's hang up 'quality of life' as a hopeless term. In: D. A. Goode (ed.) *Quality of Life for Persons with Disabilities: International Perspectives and Issues,* Cambridge, MA: Brookline Books.

Wolfensberger, W. (2000) A brief overview of Social Role Valorization, *Mental Retardation*, 38: 105–123.

Wolfensberger, W. and Glenn, L. (1973) *Program Analysis of Service Systems (PASS): A Method for the Quantitative Evaluation of Human Services*, 2nd edition, Vol. 1: *Handbook,* Vol. 2: *Field Manual,* Toronto, ONT, National Institute on Mental Retardation.

Wolfensberger, W. and Thomas, S. (1983) *PASSING (Program Analysis of Service Systems' Implementation of Normalisation Goals): Normalisation Criteria and Ratings Manual*, 2nd edition, Toronto, NIMR.

Part III

Working with people

Chapter 8

Friendships, relationships and issues of sexuality

Iain Carson and Daniel Docherty

Introduction

Most of us tend to take it for granted that friendships, relationships and the existence of social networks are a part of our lives. These can include acquaintances, work-related friendships, close friendships, family relationships, platonic personal relationships and sexual relationships. While we may often take them for granted, these are the very people that we turn to when we are sad, happy or in need of help. We share confidences with them, celebrate success together, sometimes tell them our deepest secrets. We would find life extremely difficult without them; indeed, we would probably feel very lonely and isolated. Clearly, we value them and thus feel valued in return. While many friendships and relationships are often a result of circumstances, i.e. they just happen, such 'happenings' would be unlikely had we not had the opportunity to participate in a range of social networks for example going out to play with other children, being members of extra-curricular after-school groups, going to youth clubs, and when we get older through going to college or university and entering the world of employment.

Many people with learning difficulties have been denied the opportunity to participate in such social networks and thus have few close friends. As Burke points out:

> I didn't have any close friends. I'm only just starting to have a few close friends now. Before I had no close friends at all because I'd been locked up all my life. And when you've been locked up all your life, you can't have no close friends. With that it's hard to make friends. Very hard.
>
> (Burke 2000: 110–111)

Burke is not alone; many adults with learning difficulties who spent their formative years in an institution, including residential 'special' schools, endured enforced social situations (often segregated). It could be said that non-disabled children who are educated in boarding schools have similar experiences. However, such children return to their families during periods of extensive holidays, they are allowed to leave the confines of the 'institution' and socialise with others, and, more importantly, their experience of limited social networking ends when they reach adulthood. Not so for a large number of adults with learning difficulties: even though the majority of them no longer live in institutions, the advent of community care has done little to help them in terms of developing friendships and relationships. Indeed, the *Valuing People* White Paper indicates that only 30 per cent of people with learning difficulties have a friend who doesn't have learning difficulties (DoH 2001: 20). There are many reasons for this. A large number of those who support people with learning difficulties to live within community settings often view their role from a limited perspective. They support people to maintain a standard of personal hygiene, prepare/eat food, go shopping and to a lesser extent engage in community activities. However, participation in social events often lacks variety and choice, as one man stated 'I *have* to go tenpin bowling twice a week, and I'm only allowed to go out with the staff' (Anon 2000). Why are people with learning difficulties who are supported to live in their own homes not assisted in developing friendships? Daniel Docherty, while describing his own experience later on in this chapter, alludes to one of the reasons:

> I remember a professional who used to say that learning disabled adults never grow up, they say that we're forever children.

While many of us will be shocked that a so-called 'professional' actually made this statement, this is the opinion of a number of people who support people with learning difficulties. Thus, if they perceive them to be children, they are unlikely to support them in developing friendships and relationships with adults. Some support staff view themselves as protectors of vulnerable people, and in some situations this may be true. However, we all take the risk of being hurt when we enter into a relationship and some of us need support if the relationship is unsuccessful; it is no different for people with learning difficulties. As Downer (2000: 81) states, 'I can take a risk, I can have a relationship . . . I can cry if I want to cry'. Other support staff take the view that the development of friendships and relationships might lead to sexual abuse and thus should be avoided; however, we cannot deny people the opportunity to develop personal and social networks just *in case* something undesirable happens. None the less, the issue of vulnerability and sexual abuse is a serious matter and will be discussed later in this chapter.

Services and relationships

Many services that support people with learning difficulties often feel (and are) limited in what they can provide as a result of financial constraints; it is not unusual to find one worker supporting between three and six people for an entire shift. Clearly, such situations are not conducive to the provision of person-centred support; even the most committed worker would find it difficult to support a person in developing friendships and relationships in such circumstances. A more worrying scenario, however, is the following statement made by a Canadian residential support worker:

I'm a staffperson in a residential program as well as a parent of someone with a disability. For some people I work with, I'm their only friend. What's wrong with a little hug and kiss if everyone feels good about it? There's nothing sexual in it; it's just affection.

(Melburg Schwier and Hingsburger 2000: 154)

As the authors point out, this is a clear violation of the boundaries between a service provider and a service user, and furthermore, such behaviour may well give a person with learning difficulties the impression that this is a safe activity to engage in with anyone.

Alternatives do exist; Wolfensberger (1983) suggested that citizen advocates, i.e. volunteers, were more appropriate means of support than people who were being rewarded with a salary. Certainly, a person with learning difficulties is likely to feel more valued in being supported by a voluntary 'friend' as opposed to using a service not of their choosing. However, as Goodley (2000) points out, most citizen advocacy schemes in the UK remain accountable to service systems. This is a questionable situation in relation to where the balance of power lies, i.e. the advocate is accountable to the service and the service will likely define the advocate's role – hardly an empowering situation!

One of the reasons why service providers are reluctant to encourage and support people with learning difficulties to develop friendships and relationships is because relationships can lead to sexual activity. There are two main reasons why service providers have a problem in relation to people with learning difficulties exercising their sexual rights. First, many members of staff have difficulty in separating their own moral stance from the behaviour of others, often as a result of religious convictions. McConkey and Ryan (1999) identified that staff who regularly attended places of worship held more conservative attitudes and were less supportive of sexual expression through masturbation, access to girlie magazines, one-night stands and homosexual activity. The second reason is that some members of staff quite simply do not believe that people with learning difficulties should be allowed to express themselves sexually. Daniel Docherty relates a typical scenario later in this chapter; he states that: 'a lot of staff said that we were asexual, that we couldn't have sex, and that it wasn't nice; it wasn't normal behaviour for people like us'.

There are several issues to consider here. First, why do so many members of staff think that people with learning difficulties are asexual? Basically, it has much to do with historical myths; people were portrayed as 'holy innocents', i.e. free of sexual thoughts and feelings; people have been treated as children for centuries and still are by many today; interestingly, also, the fact that children do have sexual feelings seems to be overlooked. Those who readily perpetuate these myths are thus happy to believe that sexuality does not exist. The fact that many aspects of the lives of people who have learning difficulties has moved on is not reflected in relation to their right to sexual fulfilment, quite simply because so many service providers view this whole area as a 'problem' they do not want to get involved in.

What of the statement 'you can't have sex, it isn't nice'? Isn't nice for whom? This attitude says more about the sexuality of the people holding it than it does about their views on people with learning difficulties (Rose and Jones 1994). It also highlights the power differential that still exists between service providers and service users, e.g. you can only do what I say you can do!

Policy and legal dilemmas

While many of the above staff attitudes and behaviours are a result of individual moral stances and inaccurate beliefs about the lives of people with learning difficulties, some service providers have genuine concerns about the vulnerability and/or capacity to consent to sexual relationships. This is a complex area that has been the subject of much recent debate within academic circles and government committees. In a report to the Sex Offences Review (Home Office Committee), Mencap (1999) stated that:

> the superficial impression might be that current sexual offences legislation is highly/over protective of some people with learning disabilities. The reality is that what would be rape in other cases gets downgraded to assault because the difficulty in being clear about consent reduces the potential charge to non-consensual assault rather than rape.

This demonstrates the complexity of some of the issues that need to be considered. People with learning difficulties have a right to sexual relationships, but surely they also have a right to protection from abuse (Murphy 2000). Article 8 (the right to respect for private and family life) of the Human Rights Act (1998) suggests that people with learning difficulties have the right to a sexual relationship. However, as Evans and Rodgers (2000) indicate, case law suggests that consent is crucial and thus the issue of capacity is very important. Murphy (2000: 35) summarises her understanding of the legal definition of capacity to consent to sexual relationships as:

(a) must be capable of understanding what is proposed and its implications; and

(b) must be able to exercise choice. (It is important to consider whether one party is in a position of power which will influence the ability of the other party to consent).

While referring to a recent trial (*R. v. Jenkins*) for rape, Murphy identifies that although the judge's minimal interpretation of the above definition may give people with learning difficulties the freedom to have a sexual relationship, it also suggests that anyone with a learning difficulty could not obtain a conviction of rape against an abuser. Clearly this is a dilemma that requires resolving. The Home Office (2000) recognises that the law in this area is unsatisfactory and that it is necessary to create a balance between protection and the right to a private life. It has been recommended that there should be a statutory definition of capacity to consent which reflects both knowledge and understanding of sex and its broad implications. At the time of writing, the Home Office committee recommended the adoption of a definition proposed by the Law Commission (2000: 71–72), though acknowledged that this whole area is fraught with difficulty and that further consultation was necessary.

The above dilemmas and legal complexities are ultimately the responsibility of Parliament and it is hoped that wide consultation, including people with learning difficulties themselves, will take place before the statutory framework is finalised. In the meantime, it must be recognised that people with learning difficulties have just as much need for sexual expression as the rest of society, and, where necessary, we should be supporting them to achieve this. This can include the often-difficult arena of discovering one's sexuality via emotional and physical experimentation and the hurt and trauma that often accompanies this milestone in our lives. For people employed to support people with learning difficulties, the area of personal relationships and sexuality can be complex and it is important that services have guidelines for staff (not service users) working in these areas. While there is no doubt that many people who use services are vulnerable and can be open to abuse, it needs to be recognised that service providers can also be vulnerable. However, concerns relating to the vulnerability of staff should not be at the expense of people with learning difficulties being supported to exercise their emotional, physical and sexual rights.

Ethical considerations

Many service providers find giving support of this nature challenging, unethical and in some cases impossible. This is not surprising: many readers will remember the difficulties their parents had in providing them with sex education and supporting them through the traumas of adolescence, often leaving this 'undesirable' activity to school teachers and peers. For some people, discussing such issues is just too difficult. There are many reasons for this, but this is not an appropriate forum to start trying to analyse the intricate psychological difficulties that some of us experience. However, what is important is that we feel wholly comfortable about involving ourselves in the provision of such support. Any discomfort on our part could result in a serious negative outcome for the person with learning difficulties. A more worrying scenario is where service providers who are happy to engage in such forms of support feel that it is appropriate to impose their own moral stance on the person they are supporting. An example of this is where a young man (Anon 1997) received support from an advocate to place a personal advertisement in the gay press. On receiving some responses, he showed them with real pride to his keyworker, whose immediate response was to introduce the young man to a social outlet where he might meet women. The reason being that meeting men was not 'normal'. The young man in question had spent seven years agonising over his sexual identity, and only six months previously accepted that he was gay. He now felt confused and was led to believe that he had done something wrong.

Some service providers experience dilemmas of an ethical nature when supporting people in the area of personal relationships and sexuality, these are often linked to uncertainties surrounding legal boundaries. Malin and Wilmot (2000) provide some typical examples from the work of an ethics group they were involved in, such as the man who wanted to buy pornographic materials but was physically unable to go to the shop himself, and the long-standing gay sexual relationship where staff suddenly felt uncertain about whether it was consenting or abusive. In relation to the pornography, some members of staff (male and female) felt very strongly that the man shouldn't be allowed to buy the material; others felt it was his right, depending on the degree of the pornography, and that they were duty bound to help him. One person actually approached the police force, though received little help or advice. The issues raised require some untangling: first, in relation to those who felt he shouldn't be allowed to buy the material, was it because they believed the use of pornography was morally wrong, or did they believe it would cause him harm? In either case, did they have the right to decide what was right and what was wrong or what was good for him and what was not? Second, in relation to those who felt duty bound to support the man, it is important to have a clear understanding of the law. Those of us who do not have learning difficulties rarely encounter interference in the way we choose to conduct our lives, unless of course it involves illegal activity. Why then do so many service providers feel that they have the right to regulate the choices made by some people who have learning difficulties?

In relation to the long-standing gay sexual relationship, why did it take a number of years before members of staff began to consider the possibility of exploitation? It may be because service providers have an inconsistent approach to identifying vulnerability and thus exposure to abuse. We have already acknowledged that some people with learning difficulties are more vulnerable than others and thus are more exposed to abuse.

However, vulnerability is not necessarily easily recognisable. Some service providers measure vulnerability according to the extent of a person's learning difficulties. For example, a person who has limited or no verbal communication may be considered lacking in capacity to consent to sexual relationships; this is not necessarily so. Likewise, a person who has had access to good clear sex education, is comfortable with their sexuality and has been taught how to reject unwanted attention, can still experience exploitative situations. How then do we measure vulnerability and feel able to make safe decisions in circumstances that may involve risk? Part of the problem is that many services lack adequate guidance and support for their staff. Many of those who support people with learning difficulties work in isolated situations and are frequently faced with making a wide range of decisions that may impact on the lives of those that they are supporting. Additionally, as a result of inadequate levels of staffing, and thus managers' difficulties in providing a consistent approach to cover, many people with learning difficulties find themselves being supported by people who have limited knowledge of them and are often subjected to a different support worker every other day. Perhaps more concerning is the fact, discovered in a recent survey, that 75 per cent of all staff have no relevant qualifications (Ward 1999: 1).

So, if service providers are to prove competent in assessing a person's vulnerability and thus be in a position to minimise the risk that some people with learning difficulties face, the following points must be considered in order that the people being supported are able to exercise their sexual rights with the minimum of risk:

- adequate and appropriate training needs to be provided for all staff;
- guidelines *for staff* relating to supporting people in the area of personal relationships and sexuality;
- a consistent approach to supporting people in order that the service providers actually know the people they are working with; and
- support workers are not best placed to advocate on behalf of people with learning difficulties and thus much consideration needs to be given to the issue of self-advocacy and, where appropriate, citizen advocacy.

Daniel's story, told in his own words, and which now follows, illustrates many of the points made so far.

Daniel's story

When I was a boy I only had very limited friends because I was a loner and my parents decided who my friends should be; I couldn't choose my friends. I was always inquisitive about what non-disabled children were doing, what it was like to play, what it would be like to hangout with non-disabled children. When you're hanging around disabled children you don't get the same kind of interaction; they've not got the same sort of fun in them.

I think that people used to think that I was a burden because I was disabled, I used to wonder why was I born this way? When I was a child they didn't call you disabled, they used to say I was handicapped; some people at school used to call me a 'Mong' and things like that. It's only about ten years ago that people started to say that I had learning difficulties or learning disabilities because of changes in the law, I think.

There weren't many places that you were allowed to mix with non-disabled people, I always had to go to Gateway clubs or Mencap; there was another one called Phab, it was like a youth group for disabled children and non-disabled children. These were the only places that my parents would let me go. I think that they wouldn't let me mix with non-disabled children because I wasn't ready for it, you know, didn't want to let me try to run before I could walk, they didn't want their disabled child to be led down the garden path and encouraged to do things that they wouldn't approve of. So I was never allowed to mix with non-disabled children; when I tried to they used to say 'oh no, don't talk to him, he'll try and take you to the pub or make you go to a discotheque'.

When I was a boy I only had one non-disabled friend, the rest were all disabled, and I met most of them in the institution that I was put in. The one non-disabled friend didn't stick around for long because his parents told him that he could only make friends with people like himself. We always had to play outside; our parents would never allow us to go back to each other's houses. My mother was suspicious of him for being my friend and she always wanted to ask him lots of questions; I used to think that he must have done something wrong.

When I was older, about 16 or 18, I had a wide range of friends because I didn't have my parents around to tell me who I could talk to. I had a sister who used to be quite dubious about the people I used to hang around with because she didn't want them to exploit me; it was her way of protecting me. The area where she lived had a lot of people that she didn't trust and she didn't want me to hang around with people like that; she used to say 'I don't want to see you getting hurt like you were before'. I had one non-disabled friend who used to come to the house and he used to pinch stuff, like my records; I didn't know about it until my sister told me.

When I became an adult I had a few non-disabled friends but some of them only spoke to me when they wanted something, like money. But I always used to take my sister's advice; she used to say 'don't trust a book by its cover'. So, when I meet non-disabled adults I'm always wary, I don't trust them until I get to know them. I wouldn't take them to my house or go to the pub with them, where they might buy me drinks and get me confused. If I go somewhere neutral then I can just walk off. There was this lad who used to treat me like some poor disabled person; he wasn't really my friend, he only used to see me when he had nothing else to do.

Now I've got one long-term friend, he's been my friend for fifteen years; he's a disabled person. We've got a lot in common because we're both disabled. I don't seem to stay friends with non-disabled people very long, I'm always thinking what do they want, is this genuine? They buy me dinner, what do they want in return?

I am friendly with some people who work with disabled people. They understand what it's like for disabled people because they've got knowledge about it. Most people aren't like that though, they think I'm gullible. They say things like 'you haven't got a job', 'you can't hold down a relationship', 'you should be in a day centre'. Some of them say 'you shouldn't be here, you should be in a Gateway club with your own kind'. I think that they say things like that because they think I don't know anything, I remember a professional who used to say that learning-disabled adults never grow up, they say that we're forever children. Some people take advantage of me because they think like that, like my adoptive parents. I don't want to go into detail but they took advantage in a way that they shouldn't have.

Most non-disabled people aren't going to change, if they wanted to get to know people like me they would have done it by now. Even my sister used to say 'can you catch it'? She had three kids of her own and she didn't want me hanging around them because she thought that they might catch my disability. I told her that you're born with it, it's the card you're dealt, a bit like the joker in the pack.

If I could choose my friends I'd choose people that I had something in common with, I'd look at the way they responded to me, I'd look at their body language. People put on a front sometimes, I'd want to see if they were taking me seriously rather than being patronising or sarcastic. I want them to talk to me about things that I'm interested in, not about day services and things like that. If I respect them they should respect me, but I don't think that things will change until there's full equality. Even now that I'm an adult, people still look at me as if I'm different and they don't like having eye contact with me. They're embarrassed to talk to me because they think that they're different to me, but they're not, I don't think that they are. Maybe this new Human Rights Act will stir things and make them think differently! At the moment they think of me as a reject; I just wish that they'd give me chance. If the shoe was on the other foot and disabled people had power over non-disabled people they wouldn't like it.

I think that it's hard to make friends with non-disabled people. I go to coffee bars and things, places where it's not too loud, but I don't trust some of the people that I meet, they grin at me and don't take me seriously. I very rarely make friends with anyone in these places. This man once approached me and all he did was ask me lots of questions; I don't think that he wanted to get to know me at all, just wanted to know things about me. I think that I prefer to be friends with other disabled people, non-disabled people don't know anything about our lives; they don't know what it's like to go to a special school or be in an institution or go to a day centre. I don't think that they want to know either, they're not bothered about us, sort of 'I'm alright Jack'.

The other thing I don't like about trying to make friends with non-disabled people is that they always think that I want childlike conversations! I want to talk about things like football, not 'what did you do at the day centre today' or 'did you enjoy Mencap last night'. I want to talk about what's going on outside or even the weather!

The first time I had a relationship was when I was 16 or 17, it was a sort of experiment to find out what I liked. My adoptive parents told me I could start to have friends but not a relationship. I thought I was gay and wanted to find out if I was. I was comfortable with men, but at that time I wasn't comfortable with women; I trusted men more, maybe it was because my mum left me when I was a child.

My first relationship, which was with a man of my own age was good, it made me feel good. It lasted about six months: he didn't have learning difficulties but he had a slight physical disability, he was very level headed. We used to go out to concerts together, I remember the first time, we went to see the Smiths at the Hacienda. A lot of the time we just stayed in at his house listening to music. He once took me to see Fulham, City got beat! Occasionally we'd go out for a meal at the weekend and I'd stay over at his house, but we slept in separate beds.

My adoptive mother told me that it wasn't a healthy relationship because it wasn't 'straight'; she said I could be friends with him but I couldn't have sex with him. Most people were OK about it; my sister thought it was OK, she trusted him. My adoptive father didn't like it at all, he was an ex-policeman! The only reason the relationship ended was because he had to move to London; we parted good friends.

When I was about 21 I started experimenting again. I started going out with a girl that I had known as a friend. It wasn't as good as my last relationship with a man, she had learning difficulties and was very dominant, sometimes she was aggressive towards me. It only lasted three weeks. I then developed a relationship with another girl who had learning difficulties; it became a sexual relationship and it lasted about one-and-a-half years. But then I found out that she was telling people that I wasn't good in bed. I felt very rejected at the time; it put me off having relationships with women, I couldn't trust them.

Next I had a relationship with a man who was a wheelchair user; it was a good relationship and it lasted for three years. We had our own flats but we stayed with each other quite a lot. I used to think of him as my boyfriend but I found out that he thought of me as his assistant, he used to introduce me to people as his friend. The relationship ended bad because of the way he treated me; we've never spoken since.

When I was 25 I was going to college doing what they called a special needs course; reading and writing it was. It was there I met Trish: at that time we were mostly friends and this lasted until I left college. Meeting Trish made me realise that I was bisexual rather than gay. I think that the relationship didn't develop because her parents didn't want it to happen. When I left college I didn't see her again for about two or three years; I missed her a lot and used to send her letters, but I found out that her mother kept them. Then I met her again at People First. I was really pleased to see her but it was strange because we had to behave as if we were just friends, even though we wanted it to be more. I think it was difficult because staff at People First thought I was gay.

After about three months things with Trish got very serious and she started staying at my house. The support workers were worried because she was never at home; they kept saying that they wanted to know where she was staying. On New Year's Eve we got engaged, I proposed to her and she said yes! We went out to buy a ring and she ran away, she wasn't sure if I thought she was worth it. Most of our problems came from Trish's parents; they kept sticking their nose in and said I wasn't suitable. They thought I was a liar and they said I had 'mental schizophrenia', so it's been hard for us. Everybody else was really good; they encouraged us to have a relationship because they thought we looked happy together. Except Trish's support worker, who said we'd be better off on our own and not have a relationship.

I miss my sister; she died about two years ago. She used to support me with my friendships and relationships; she was like a mother figure. I remember when people used to bully me; she always stood up for me.

Trish and I decided to live together about six months ago. The staff at People First are helping us with things like getting Direct Payments and sorting the flat out. We're not getting married yet, maybe in three or four years; we'd like to have a baby but that won't be for a long time. Our relationship is strong and it's blossoming, we both know how we feel. I think she's wonderful, she makes me happy; she's very strong for a disabled woman. I think we'll be very happy in our relationship but I think that Trish will need to stand up to her mum.

When I was about 16 or 17 I remember members of staff telling me that I couldn't have sex or even masturbate. They told me that masturbating was wrong, they used to say that it wasn't good for me and that I'd go blind and get hairy hands; maybe they were being over-protective. The thing is I haven't had very many sexual relationships, didn't want them because of what happened to me when I was a child: I need to trust people. Anyway, the staff used to say that people like me, people with learning difficulties, shouldn't have relationships, especially sexual relationships. A lot of staff said that we were asexual, that we couldn't have sex, and that it wasn't nice; it wasn't normal behaviour for people like us. They expected us to just sit around watching television all the time or doing nought; they thought that our brain couldn't cope with sexual relationships. Some staff said that because our brains were different we couldn't think for ourselves and that we always copied other people, they said that this might lead to sexual abuse. My sister used to tell me that it was all right to kiss but that I mustn't do anything else, 'remember what happened when you were a kid' she used to say, she said it would happen again.

I was once caught by a member of staff doing something in the bedroom; I was on my own and it was private, but they always used to walk in without knocking to see what I was doing. When they caught me masturbating they said 'you shouldn't be doing that, it's not nice, it's not allowed'. I told them that they shouldn't come into my bedroom, but they said they had the power to do this in case I was harming myself; I thought that they might be right and that maybe sex was dirty.

Some staff used to say that I shouldn't have sex because I would get abused, but I know when something's nice and when it isn't. The first time that I had sex was with a woman who had learning difficulties; it was nice, a nice feeling in my body, but it didn't feel nice in my head, I still thought that it was dirty. I remember once when I went out for a drink in the gay village this (non-disabled) man invited me back to his house for a cup of coffee. I thought that this was OK because I just wanted to meet someone for a chat, but when we got there he took all my clothes off, even though I said I don't want that. I know that I should have just said no, but at the time I didn't know how to. It's not that I didn't want to have sex with someone like him, he liked me and I liked him, but I just wasn't in the mood for things like that.

Most of my sexual relationships have been with disabled people; I think it's because we're both on the same wavelength, we've got something in common and we know what it's like to be put down by non-disabled people. I have had a sexual relationship with a non-disabled person, like the one I mentioned earlier. It was all right for the first year, but after that he wasn't very nice, he told my father what we were doing together, so I fell out with him and now we don't speak.

When I was younger I thought that sex was interesting, but as I got older I used to think that it was dirty and that it got me into trouble. I always met the wrong sort of people and, because at that time I didn't like to say no, people used to think that I was one of these people who was always at it! But now, I only have sex when I want it because I don't want to get into trouble with the wrong sort of people, like the people who used to take money from me; most of my sexual relationships have been with men. Maybe I should have taken my sister's advice and only kissed people, but I wouldn't have been happy about that, I would have regretted not having sex.

If I was asked to give advice (about sex) to a young man with learning difficulties, I would say take it one step at a time, don't dive in with both feet because you don't know who the person is, it could be a mass murderer. I would tell them, make sure you get a lot of information, a lot of advice about safe sex and HIV, and if it was with a woman, about diseases and pregnancy. I would tell them to do something I haven't always done, use your own judgement and don't have sex with them after one meeting; you have to meet them loads and loads of times before you have sex. Even if you know that kissing them is nice, you should get to know them and make friends with them first: start going out on dates with them and try to get your head clear about them because lots of people want to exploit men and women who have learning difficulties. I think that members of staff should support people and give them advice, but whatever you tell the staff should be kept confidential, they should only tell the manager if it's something serious, like getting someone pregnant, but not if you want some condoms. I don't think that staff should be writing in their records about our sex lives, it shouldn't be allowed.

I remember when Trish said that she was leaving her house to live with me, the leader of the house asked her if she was having sex. A few days afterwards this member of staff said 'What are you having sex for? You're not to have it.' Trish told me that the staff wanted to have a meeting about us having sex, I think that they wanted to make sure that we were both being safe because I'd been with men. They said that Trish was vulnerable and that they didn't want me to leave her in the lurch, but I wouldn't do that, she's too precious. I do window shop sometimes, but I don't buy because it's expensive!

The worst sexual experience I've ever had was with that guy I was talking about earlier, the one who used to treat me like his assistant. I don't think that he had any real feelings for me, it was just about having sex when he wanted it, not when I wanted it, and if I didn't do it he would go mad. I think that my best experience is what I've got now with Trish.

What needs to change?

Before I finish, I'd like to tell you about the four things I'd like to see change:

- There should be some sort of commission group to look at relationships and sex for people who have learning difficulties, but there should be a certain percentage of learning-disabled people in the group. It should be their job to change the law so that things were equal for us like everybody else.

- There should be someone employed to give advice about sexual health issues, like HIV, different kinds of relationships, gay or lesbian, bisexual and them sort of things. It should be there all the time when we think we need it, not when staff think we've got needs. Also, it shouldn't just be things in writing, they should have pictures and tapes and things like that.
- There should be some kind of parents and carers' group but it should be chaired by someone with a disability. It could be like a workshop and you ask the parents and carers what they see as the problems and the hurdles; it would be a way of learning for them.
- There should be sexual awareness training for staff and for people with learning difficulties.

These are the points that I would look at because I don't think that people who are learning disabled are going to go back into hiding. We're always going to have sexual urges; if we're not allowed to masturbate, if services keep saying 'this is a bad thing, this is not good for you', things will stay hard for us. As somebody with a learning disability who's got a partner, I'd say its not been easy; it's been hard. I think that things have got to change, quickly and fast, but I don't think that staff are bothered, they'll just keep taking us to the day centre, it's not fair.

Conclusion

It is clear that many people with learning difficulties are not being supported to develop friendships and relationships, and even less are being supported to exercise their sexual rights. Consequently, they continue to experience far greater social and emotional isolation than most other members of society. *Valuing People* (DoH 2001: 23) has stated that Rights, Independence, Choice and Inclusion are 'at the heart of the Government's proposals' in relation to improving the lives of people who have learning difficulties. They have also more specifically stated that: 'good services will help people with learning disabilities develop opportunities to form relationships, including ones of a physical and sexual nature'. However, they also indicate that: 'helping people sustain friendships is consistently shown as being one of the greatest challenges faced by learning disability services'.

This is one of the challenges that service providers are simply going to have to overcome if they genuinely want to end the discrimination that people with learning difficulties are currently experiencing.

The White Paper (DoH 2001: 98) has stated that by 2005 50 per cent of all front-line staff should have achieved at least an NVQ Level Two Certificate in Working with People who have Learning Disabilities. However, it is unlikely that training at this level will equip staff with the necessary expertise to support people in this area. Service managers may need to consider the provision of specialist in-house staff training if they are to successfully achieve the Government's proposals. In relation to guidelines for staff supporting people in this area, many services already have these in place. However, producing guidelines is not enough; the information contained within such policy documents needs to be disseminated to all staff and training relating to their implementation should be an integral part of a rolling programme of staff development.

The White Paper (DoH 2001: 47) has set a target of at least one citizen advocacy group existing in each Local Authority area by 2004. This will go some way towards enabling people with learning difficulties to develop friendships and relationships and is more appropriate than support workers advocating on behalf of the people they work with.

However, citizen advocates, even those with the best of intentions, will to some extent exert control over the lives of the individuals they are advocating on behalf of. It is therefore important that greater consideration is given to the funding and development of local self-advocacy groups, the preferred choice of many people with learning difficulties, because, in the words of Gary Bourlet (1988: 21): 'self-advocacy enables us to make choices and make our decisions and control the way that our lives should be made'.

So, if we truly want to enable people with learning difficulties to develop friendships and have relationships, including ones of a physical and sexual nature, we need to start asking the people themselves how best we can enable them to achieve this.

References

Anon (1997) *Personal Story of a Service User*, Greater Manchester, Unpublished.
Anon (2000) *Personal Story of a Service User*, Greater Manchester, Unpublished.
Bourlet, G. (1988) A share of the action for consumers, *Community Living*, April: 20–21.
Burke, P. (2000) It is true. I know it is. In: D. Goodley (2000) *Self-advocacy in the Lives of People with Learning Difficulties*, Buckingham, Open University Press.
Department of Health (2001) *Valuing People: A New Strategy for Learning Disability for the 21st Century*, London, The Stationery Office.
Downer, J. (2000) Ask self-advocates. In: D. Goodley (2000) *Self-advocacy in the Lives of People with Learning Difficulties*, Buckingham, Open University Press.
Evans, A. and Rodgers, M. E. (2000) Protection for whom? The right to a sexual or intimate relationship, *Journal of Learning Disabilities*, 4 (3): 237–245.
Goodley, D. (2000) *Self-advocacy in the Lives of People with Learning Difficulties*, Buckingham, Open University Press.
Home Office (2000) *Setting the Boundaries*, Vol. 1, London, The Stationery Office.
The Law Commission (2000) Vulnerable people. In: The Home Office *Setting the Boundaries*, Vol. 1, London, The Stationery Office, p. 71.
McConkey, R. and Ryan D. (1999) *Staff Attitudes to Sexuality and People with Intellectual Disabilities*, Newtownabbey, University of Ulster. Online:
   http://www.ulst.ac.uk/faculty/shse/research/cnr/ldisability/ld_articpapers/7_17b.htm
Malin, N. A. and Wilmot, S. (2000) An ethical advisory group in a learning disability service – Members' views on outcomes, *Journal of Learning Disabilities*, 4 (4): 333–342.

Meldburg Schwier, K. and Hingsburger, D. (2000) *Sexuality – Your Sons and Daughters with Intellectual Disabilities*, London, Jessica Kingsley Publishers.

Mencap (1999) Submission to the Sex Offences Review, cited in Home Office (2000) *Setting the Boundaries*, Vol. 1, London, The Stationery Office.

Murphy, G. (2000) Capacity to consent to sexual relationships in people with learning disabilities, *British Journal of Learning Disabilities*, 29(1): 35.

Rose, J. and Jones, C. (1994) Working with parents. In: A. Craft [ed.] *Practice issues in Sexuality and Learning Disabilities*, London, Routledge.

Ward, F. (1999) *Modernising the Social Care Workforce – the First National Training Strategy for England: Supplementary Report on Learning Disability*, Leeds, TOPPS England.

Wolfensberger, W. (1983) *Reflections on the Status of Citizen Advocacy*, Toronto, NIMR

Chapter 9

Social inclusion and people with profound and multiple disabilities

Reality or myth?

Sarah Rooney

Introduction

The segregation and social isolation of people with learning difficulties has long been the subject of debate. Increased insight and awareness of people's lives have resulted in a realisation that people with learning difficulties have the right to learn, work, live and play alongside their non-disabled counterparts, and that most actively desire this for themselves (Wertheimer 1996; McIntosh and Whittaker 2000; O'Brien and Lyle O'Brien 2000).

This chapter aims to critically examine issues which affect how people, who as a result of their additional physical impairments are referred to as having 'complex needs', become involved in ordinary activities and develop personal relationships. The roles that contemporary initiatives, such as person-centred planning, direct payments and supported living, have in enabling people with complex support needs to lead less segregated lives and work towards what has been euphemistically referred to as an 'ordinary life' will be explored.

Current services

As other chapters have illustrated, despite improvements in the way learning disabilities services are delivered many people with learning difficulties spend their days in impersonal day services, large group homes, or remain at home with their family, receiving little or no service at all (Fruin 1998; King's Fund 1999).

As Wertheimer (1996) observed, 'the lifestyles of most people with learning disabilities are still largely dictated by services. Where they live, what they do, who they live with, where they go and who supports them are all determined by paid "specialist" services' (p. 2).

As a result of using 'specialist' services people with learning difficulties have to comply with established routines (Edge 2001). These are designed to ensure the smooth running of a particular establishment. Many day centres, for example, operate around timetables, which limit the flexibility to support individual interests and aspirations. They do, however, offer respite care for families, limited occupational activities and a meeting place for friends. In this sense it could be argued that services have an important role to play in providing support to both people with learning difficulties and their carers. In reality learning disability services often perpetuate ideas of separateness and difference, where individual needs are sacrificed to the demands of staff availability and reducing budgets. (Simons 1999). Despite the rhetoric that surrounds the improvement and modernisation of care services, it is still apparent that 'principles are weak when faced with long standing rationing of services' (Felce *et al.* 1998).

In this new century it is more commonplace for people with learning difficulties to be part of society through attending college, gaining employment and living in supported housing. Nevertheless, many remain marginalised on the periphery of community life. As the Scottish Executive (2000) in their report *The Same As You?* concluded, it appears that, 'far from supporting the principles of an "ordinary life" . . . all too often services act to maintain exclusion' (p. 25).

Although the wholesale 'warehousing' of people with learning difficulties is declining, institutional custody in a smaller, and more insidious form, exists within local communities. The creation of 'new' institutions can be seen in all service sectors. Discreet education provision creates educational ghettos within mainstream opportunities (Dowson 1998). Day services cater for groups of people too large for individual hopes and aspirations to be addressed. All too often those living within supported houses remain 'house bound' as low staffing levels prevent them from going out. In short, as Hatton and Emerson (1996), McIntosh and Whittaker (1998) and Simons and Watson (1999b) suggest, there is little evidence to demonstrate that living *in* the community ensures that people with learning difficulties become *part of it*.

Services and people with complex needs

Consequently, while people with learning difficulties are more visible in our local neighbourhoods than they were thirty years ago, many still lead lonely, isolated lives. This is true for many people with learning difficulties, but it is particularly so for those who Morris (1999) sensitively describes as having 'continuing health care needs and/ or multiple impairments' (p. 7). She further suggests that although professionals use the label 'complex health and support needs', it is not the individuals' needs that are complex, but the lengths they have to go to to obtain appropriate help.

As well as having particular support needs, many of these people face numerous challenges when attempting to communicate with those around them (Bradley 1998). It is crucial, therefore, that efforts are made to ensure that the 'voice' of each individual is heard and their wishes are noted. As McIntosh and Whittaker (2000) have asserted, it is difficult to be 'part of a community if [you] are unable to communicate and interact. Communication is the precursor to social activity. It underpins confidence, equality, empowerment and friendship' (p. 17). Bradley (1998), in agreement, says that 'communication is the rock' upon which all relationships and social activities rest (p. 50). Although many people with complex needs do not use speech, each person has their own unique way of getting their message across. Understanding the wants of someone who does not use verbal language, however, takes time and involves significant commitment to the individual (Caldwell 1996; Smull 1996; Caldwell and Stevens 1998).

As the numbers of people with complex needs using services appears to be increasing, careful thought should be given to the manner in which these are organised and apportioned. The Department of Health observed that a growing number of younger people with higher levels of disability are coming into adult services via the school system (DoH 1998a). Moreover, as a result of recent advances in health care, people with profound disabilities are living longer (DoH 2000), thus increasing numbers of older people requiring greater levels of support.

Concerns: questions for consideration

Experience gained supervising student placements and providing training for a range of independent and social services has highlighted many issues that relate to the support of people who have complex needs. Concerns repeatedly voiced in training confirm the disillusionment often felt by paid and unpaid carers. The following examples illustrate some of the dilemmas confronting those delivering learning disability services or providing individualised care.

A highly motivated and dedicated student abandoned her training and employment within learning disability services in her final year of study. After several years of working within a large hostel she had looked forward to moving to an ordinary house with three women with whom she had built good relationships. The physical move was planned in a thoughtful way and the women concerned were involved from the outset in choosing their new home, its décor and furnishings. Although they had no choice about the people they lived with, the women were delighted that hostel staff were going to support them in their new home.

All went well, until it became apparent that the staffing levels in the house were simply too low. The women all used wheelchairs, and to have any real quality of life, they needed at least two staff to work in their home during the day. The social service department refused to provide 'double cover'. As a result, the women, who had been compulsorily retired from the day centre, never left the house. It was impossible to take people out either collectively or as individuals. The situation became so appalling that the student had to do the household shopping in her own time, because it was simply not possible for her to leave the house during her work shift. She coped in this situation for six months, during which time the women she supported remained housebound. The staffing situation deteriorated, as the original staff left and were replaced by a string of agency workers.

The student, disillusioned by the concept of 'community care' and how badly it had let the women she worked with down, changed career paths completely. The large, dilapidated hostel had, in its own way, provided opportunities for wider relationships and greater community involvement and continuity of support. This had been exchanged for an attractive, sterile prison, which was expected to run with the same staff-ratio as the hostel, but ultimately provided less scope for personalised support. This example supports research undertaken by Heller *et al.* (1999), who discovered that although people living in community housing often had greater integration than those living in care or nursing homes, this was dependent on staff supporting the social inclusion of the people they worked with. Emerson *et al.* (1999) indicate that the engagement in community or household activities of people with complex needs is dependent on individualised practical support.

The difficulties related to staffing levels and groupings of people are not restricted to residential provision. Many workers have spoken of their frustrations and inability to address basic support needs within localised, smaller day services. Developments in daytime opportunities for more able people has meant that 'the average dependency of users remaining in centres [is] increasing' (Fruin 1998: 24). It has been noted that there has been a growth in day services places for people with greater and more complex needs (DoH 1999). This trend is in danger of creating locally based 'special care units' or ghettos of more severely impaired people, as those who are more able are supported towards greater independence, or are simply assessed as no longer needing a service!

Felce (1999, cited by Simons and Watson 1999a) had similar concerns about these changes in learning disability services and the tendency to congregate people with severe impairments together. He noted the greater a person's support needs, the more likely they were to be assembled into 'pathologically defined' groups of people and be 'excluded from all but a limited range of options' (p. 23).

Day service staff frequently expressed concerns about the way they were prevented from meeting individual people's personal care and health needs. This was a far greater concern than enabling a person to engage in an activity that reflected their personal interest within either the day service or the community. Staffs' inability to provide for a person's basic fundamental rights such as assisting them with a drink, to eat their lunch or to change the incontinence pad that had in some cases been in place all day, leads to far greater distress for all involved.

Similar worries were voiced at a regional People First Conference. Both people with learning difficulties and those who supported them spoke about the numerous pitfalls encountered when trying to provide individual support. An illustration of this was the frequently reported practice of having to take all the people who lived in one house to an individuals' doctor or dentist appointment or, in an emergency, to the hospital casualty department. The above accounts endorse Ward's (2000) thoughts when she concludes that 'service opportunities for people with profound and complex needs must be expanded. There is such evidence that these groups of people are currently poorly served in all areas' (p. 34).

The Department of Health White Paper *Valuing People* (2001) responds to these issues and says that 'services are often not tailored to the needs and abilities of the individual (p. 2) and that progress towards modernisation has 'been too slow'. Its findings also indicate that 'the most severely disabled people often receive the poorest service' (p. 77).

It may appear pessimistic and counterproductive to dwell on the difficulties that exist within services, rather than focus on positive approaches to delivery. Personal experience, however, has shown that innovative and creative approaches are somewhat thin on the ground, despite a reported increased commitment to the promotion of self-determination and better standards of living for people with learning difficulties and a greater awareness of the concept of interdependence. As a trainer, I have often been accused of 'not telling it as it really is' when providing examples of thoughtful and person-centred approaches. Idealistic young students, experiencing service provision, become disillusioned when faced with the reality of the situation. Parents, and staff working within services, are convinced that my views are those of 'an off-the-wall academic' who does not understand the concerns and hardships that face those involved on a day-to-day basis. Ward (2000) has written extensively about the challenges that confront parents and carers. She identifies major concerns related to the way services are delivered. A family carer echoed Ward's misgivings when he said 'if you only comment on the good things, bad practice gets away with it'.

It appears that those who depend on or work within learning disability services have concerns that mirror Fruin's view when he argues that services

> whether residential or day, . . . are becoming more responsive to individual needs and providing greater choice. But SSDs have further work to do before the services they provide, arrange with others or commission measure fully up to the service principles which now underpin development plans.
>
> (Fruin 1998:9)

A personal perspective

To help me explore the issues that affect the inclusion of people with complex needs, from a personal perspective, I approached a family to assist in the writing of this chapter. This was important, because as Sanderson (1998b) acknowledges, it is the family who knows the person best. The Norman family consists of mum and dad, Bernadette and Roger, and their two sons, Karl and Matthew. Bernadette and Roger have attended training courses and impressed both myself and other participants with their knowledge, and commitment to, not only their own sons, but also other people with learning difficulties.

Karl

Karl is 22 years old and lives at home with his parents and younger brother Matthew. He has a girlfriend of four years called Yvonne. Karl enjoys socialising with people. He particularly enjoys going to the pub for a drink or going out for a meal. He loves music and dancing and is always the last to leave any party. Karl also has a rare disabling medical condition. This condition has no name; tests have shown that only one other person in the world has this condition, his brother Matthew.

Karl's disability means that he is unable to support himself. He uses a special seat in a wheelchair; has little or no speech, but uses body language and Makaton signs to make himself understood. He has numerous medical problems and deteriorating health. He uses a day service for five days a week, where he has one-to-one support. He also has one-to-one support at home for sixty-and-a-half hours a week from paid staff. His parents care for him for the rest of the week.

Matthew

Matthew is 20 years old. He lives at home with his parents and older brother Karl. Matthew is a quieter man than his brother. He prefers to sit silently in a group of people until he feels relaxed in their company. Once he has gained confidence he is very outgoing. He likes to party, and particularly enjoys dancing and singing. He has a girlfriend called Emma. Matthew also enjoys nature, particularly animals. He is 'into cars' in a big way and is desperate to drive a racing car.

Matthew also has a rare disabling condition. The only other person known to have this condition in the world is his older brother Karl. Matthew requires a specially made chair inside his wheelchair to support him. He has some word sounds and loves to hold conversations, although this can be very frustrating for him. Matthew uses Makaton signs and body language to communicate. He has many medical problems and deteriorating health.

Matthew attends a day service for five days a week, where he has one-to-one support. He is supported at home for sixty-five-and-a-half hours a week by paid staff and by his parents for the remaining hours.

Roger

Roger is a 46-year-old married man, with two sons. Prior to being made redundant three years ago, he worked as a senior instructor at a dental hospital. He now has his own transport business specialising in offering a service to people who use wheelchairs.

Roger spends most of his non-paid working time caring for his sons. Roger's entire life revolves around his family and issues of care. As a result of this he is constantly tired. The continual fight for services for his sons increasingly frustrates him.

Bernadette

Bernadette is 48 years old. She is married with two sons. She is a qualified nurse and a child care officer. She no longer has paid employment, as she cares for her two sons. She takes responsibility for all tasks that relate to the employment of Karl and Matthew's home support staff.

Over the years Bernadette has supported both sons at home and has fought for the right to care for them. This has resulted in her acquiring a reputation from some providers of services. Although the family no longer uses these services, her name and reputation live on!

The permanent fight for responsive services has worn Bernadette down and the battle continues in order to ensure that the right ones are in place. Bernadette's days are spent caring for her two sons. She would now like to take a 'back seat', but is not confident that Karl and Matthew would have the same level and quality of care should she and Roger withdraw. Her concerns do not necessarily relate to what services her sons use, but to having the right level and calibre of people to support them in their home and community.

The issues

Our conversations focused on the following aspects that have direct relevance to Karl and Matthew being part of their local and wider community:

- what is available?;
- what is not available?;
- supported living;
- person-centred planning, direct payments;
- the role of the parent as an advocate; and
- inclusion.

What is available?

As previously stated, Matthew and Karl receive a day service from Monday to Friday. This has been achieved because 'we fought for it and also the one-to-one support that Karl and Matthew have at the day centre – they are the only people to have this'. Bernadette and Roger feel that they have good relationships with the staff at the day service and that they *listen* and respond to their concerns.

Although Karl and Matthew use a day service that is essentially building based, the one-to-one support they each have enables them to go out when they wish. Bernadette and Roger said that if this were not so, they would have concerns about their sons 'going to the same place every day'.

Karl and Matthew individually have a team of three support workers who know them well and support them in the day centre at different times of the week. Getting to know Karl and Matthew means learning how to communicate with them through Makaton signs and interpretation of body language and facial expressions. This ensures continuity, but also allows for planned change. Each support worker has been introduced on a gradual basis. Having a team of people also means that any time off can be covered 'so there are no harrowing stories of no care'. Again it was emphasised that the 'service listens' to what Karl and Matthew want, as well as parental concerns.

In the early 1990s, the local Social Service Department asked the family to pilot Individual Living Funding as a means of providing support at home. This funding was used to buy in care for Karl and Matthew. Initially the money was used to pay for one support worker for an hour in the morning before school and for two hours after school. Funding increased when Bernadette had a hysterectomy. This enabled the family to employ two people to work for the hours outlined above. Social Services, through their community care budgets, funded the difference between the Independent Living Fund monies and the support costs. Some home-based weekend support was offered at this point.

Shortly after this time Bernadette injured her back in a road traffic accident. The injuries resulted in her being unable to lift. The level of support was extended until 10 p.m. for most but not all evenings. As a result Roger had to lift his sons on his own through the night. Constant lifting caused severe damage to his back, resulting in surgery to remove several discs. Social Services helped the family through this crisis by increasing the funding into the home to include overnight staffing. Bernadette explained that 'Social services have responded on a sliding scale, increasing and withdrawing funding according to need'. The family then decided to use the funding they received via the Independent Living Fund and the Social Services to recruit and employ their own staff, rather than using agency workers.

As the level of funding for home support has not risen since the early 1990s, recruitment of home staff is becoming increasingly difficult. Bernadette reported that the hourly rate paid then was a 'good wage', now it is barely above the statutory minimum. Staff have commented that they would 'get more pay in other services, and even better in local supermarkets!' Higher rates of pay would result in a reduction of the level of support that Karl and Matthew currently receive.

The family have a break from one another roughly one weekend a month. Initially Karl and Mathew used residential services away from the home, but because of their particular health care needs it became more appropriate for them to remain in their own specially adapted home. The additional organisation and planning required prior to a stay away from home made short-term breaks arduous. Extra support is put into the home every fifth weekend to enable Bernadette and Roger to get away for a couple of nights. This care effectively allows them to leave the house from Friday night until Sunday evening, but if an emergency arises they are asked to return home. The family has a community nurse they see about twice a month and a social worker they can contact when 'they have a problem'.

What is not available?

Karl and Matthew do not use the leisure or employment services available locally to other young disabled people. Bernadette believes this is because 'services are frightened by their needs'. They were denied entry to one 'special' club because of the 'risk' this involved. Others accepted Karl and Matthew as long as they brought their personal support workers with them, which made them feel 'different'. Interestingly, Karl and Matthew have fewer problems socialising with their support workers in 'ordinary' club settings than they do in segregated ones.

Now that Karl and Matthew are older and adult services have 'inherited them and the family set up', pressure is being exerted on the family to change to direct payment. They have concerns that direct payment will not be as flexible as previous funding arrangements. Bernadette commented that 'there is too much demarcation between health and social services. It should be a package. At the moment a person is split up into bits. There seems to be discussion around what is a health need and what is a social need and who pays for what?' She has been told that direct payments cannot be used to provide for a person's health needs. Karl and Matthew are now tube fed and, at times, require oxygen to help them breath. These tasks are classed as 'health needs'. Bernadette argued that 'if you can't feed them, they cannot go out – so isn't that a social need?'

The changes in funding that have accompanied Karl and Matthews' move into adult services has resulted in a decrease in the level of their personal support. The local health authority refuses to pay for regular support at night. The family often waits six weeks for assistance with the care that Karl and Matthew require twenty-four hours a day. Short-term care is funded 'as a favour' through the local health service learning disability budget. Because of cuts in these budgets, Bernadette and Roger have been told that 'they should be grateful for what they get'.

The family commented that because they believe that 'respite within services is not suitable for Karl and Matthew' they actually get less support at home than they would if they used a residential home for short-term breaks. They are also acutely aware that choosing to care for Karl and Matthew at home, both in the short term and long term provokes much criticism. Bernadette said:

> People say you should let go, but you can't let go until you know the level of service is right. We've fought for this for twenty-three years. It's the level of care I would want for myself. I would not want to be left to lie in a wet bed.

Relationships and inclusion

Despite the barriers to specialist leisure services Karl and Matthew have good community links. Support workers from the day service help them participate in local activities and visit places that interest them. They have girlfriends they met through college. Like most young men Karl and Matthew invite them back to their home and go out for meals and other dates together. Unlike other young people they require support from their parents and personal support workers to do this. Karl and Matthew also attend church and drink in a range of pubs.

Bernadette and Roger have been determined that their sons' impairments should not prevent them from getting involved. They enjoy:

- holidays abroad – travelling by both sea and air;
- outdoor pursuits, e.g. assault courses, sailing, horse riding;
- shopping – in up-market shopping malls; and

- charity events, for example, a 'Challenge' to get to Dublin and back for only ten pounds.

When asked if they felt that their sons were 'included' in community life, Bernadette said yes they were, but this resulted from 'a lot of work and funding'. She reflected that it was:

> not a natural inclusion, it's a manufactured one and therefore the idea of inclusion is a myth – but it can happen, it could. Fairy tales, you know, can have happy endings.

Karl and Matthew both have acquaintances they have met through the pub, church and the Dublin challenge. Although people chat to them in social situations, that is the sum total of the level of involvement. They say that their true friends are disabled people. Bernadette and Roger were sceptical about the concept of natural supports.

> Over the years many people have been involved in Karl's and Matthew's lives, but none have stayed – people make a short-term commitment, but it doesn't last.

Advocacy and person-centred planning

Bernadette and Roger have always used person centred approaches to plan for the support their sons receive, although they were never aware of the term. Having individualised support is at the heart of whatever services or funding they have fought for. They pioneered 'supported living' long before it became a recognised alternative to residential care. Both, however, are conscious that others might say that they speak for, instead of on behalf of Karl and Matthew. Bernadette says that 'if Karl and Matthew could speak they would get a lot more'.

She is also aware that the path she and Roger tread is a difficult one:

> Karl would say I've ruined his life – all the bad things have been caused by me. Without us to fight for them, Karl and Matthew would have been forgotten by people. I'm not sure if that is the role of an advocate. I hope that as an advocate I always fought for what is right for them, but it's not always been right for us, and who takes over from us if we are not there?

Being a friend, advocate, parent and organiser of the care that Karl and Matthew receive has not been an easy option. Bernadette and Roger reflected that it has been a 'struggle, no time for yourself. It would be nice not to be thought of as a pain – or its them again or not that . . . bitch!'

Conclusions

The White Paper focuses on promoting independence and social inclusion. It has a huge agenda. The major review of services that will take place over the next decade, and beyond, will undoubtedly consider the way services are assisting people to develop relationships and have some control over their lives (Poxton *et al.* 2001). To support people with complex needs to have at least some of the experiences in life most of us take for granted it is crucial that the following issues are taken account of.

Quality of life

Johnstone (1998: 59) has stated that quality of life is a 'multidimensional concept'. Although the evaluation of another person's life is subjective, we should make sure that people's health needs are met and they have good housing, an income and the opportunity to make relationships and engage in activities of their choice.

It is also important to consider what monitoring exists to ensure a person's safety. O'Brien and Lyle O'Brien (1996) commented that 'people with significant disabilities cannot take even the most basic human and civil rights for granted'. They have also argued that even those who have 'good supports and opportunities can slip into isolation, neglect and abuse' (p. 5). As support becomes more individualised and community based this is difficult to monitor and control.

Researchers continually seek ways to measure the 'quality of life concept' (Felce and Perry 1995; Rose 1998; and see Chapter 7). The reality is we will never *truly know* how often a person sits alone in front of a TV screen, or on a separate table in a restaurant while paid workers chat together. Or how often they are pushed around the supermarket whilst the shopping is done for, not with them? It seems almost an impossible task to ensure that people are 'saved' from being lonely in their own homes, forsaken within poorly staffed day services or from being onlookers, rather than participants of community life. As Holman and Collins (1998) point out, 'having the right staff is a hugely important matter . . . having the right or wrong staff affects every aspect of people's lives and the control or lack of it, that they have' (p. 233).

The Department of Health's (1998b) White Paper *Modernising Social Services* states that 'individual practitioners should be personally accountable for their own standards of conduct and practice' (p. 36). However, it offers no guarantees that workers will act in a responsible and sensitive way, or that they have a clear understanding of what this means. People with complex needs are easy targets for lazy or exploitative staff. If asked to monitor their own practice, abusive staff will simply record what they think their managers want to read, which may not be an accurate record of what has been done!

The Human Rights Act 1998, which came into force in October 2000, or the Care Standards Act 2000 to be implemented in 2002, will do little to 'police' the emotional and social neglect of people, which so often occurs, and is not evidenced by bruises or physical scars. Performance indicators can never truly divulge how often a person who cannot easily complain is talked to or what social interaction takes place. In-depth recording of a person's social engagement takes time, and workers simply cannot fit any more into their day. It is easy to jot down that someone went to the pub, or for a walk, but it is far more time consuming and demanding to think about, and record exactly what went on.

Continuity of support

This is especially important for those people with complex needs who use alternative methods of communication. The need to develop close relationships in order to interpret individual wishes and fears has been well documented (Sanderson *et al.* 1997). The development of a stable, professional workforce against a background of no contracts, poor wages, little opportunity for staff training, long working hours, and often lonely working conditions seems problematic. As Cervi (1996) has indicated, when employment conditions for workers are poor, then it is likely that people who use services have an inferior standard of care.

The White Paper makes recommendations for staff training and development; however, it says little that will encourage workers to stay in people's lives through improved conditions of employment.

Reliable dependent advocacy

As a result of the Normans' continued fight for improved support for Karl and Matthew, the quality of service they have received might be judged to be of a good standard. Their situation embodies many of the principles of good 'supported living' in that they live in their own home. Mum and dad have a flat above their premises. Karl and Matthew have some control over where they live, in that they remain in their local neighbourhood, in their own home, they invite their girlfriends to their house, they make everyday choices. They choose their support workers with their parents' guidance. None of this would have been achieved without Bernadette and Rogers' perseverance. Their role echos Dowson's (1999) observations when he says that:

> many people with learning difficulties, as a result of their impairment and their devalued status, will need help from other people. In the language of services they have the role of 'advocates', but they may see themselves simply as family and friends.
>
> (p 9)

There are, however, many people with complex needs who do not have anyone to speak for them. As a consequence they are often overlooked; they remain unaware that they have a right to control, or change, their lives. They cannot conceive of being asked the kind of question posed by Sanderson (1998a) when she enquired 'What can we do together to achieve a better life for you now and in the future?' (p. 163). Opportunities for citizen advocacy could make a significant difference to the way people with complex disabilities are helped to have their opinions heard. The White Paper recognises that advocacy has been unevenly developed across the country, due to insecure funding and conflicts of interest, but insists 'this must change' (p. 46) (see Chapter 10 for a wider discussion on advocacy).

Variety of support

Natural supports may be the way to create greater opportunities for individualised help (O'Brien and Lyle O'Brien, 2000). Effective use of community networks widens the scope of a person's care package and develops their relationship circles. To fully develop this concept, service providers will be challenged to find ways to persuade volunteers of the value of getting *and staying* involved.

Direct Payments

The Community Care (Direct Payments) Act 1996 gave Local Authorities the power to make direct cash payments for community care to those who need services. By giving the consumer of services financial control the intention is to promote independence and social inclusion by offering opportunities for personalised support.

As the White Paper explains, the success of Direct Payments for people with learning disabilities depends on good services. The difficulty that exists for people with complex needs is that there is little reliable information available to them. Unfortunately, many carers, or their social workers, have never heard of Direct Payments. Those parents who are well informed have mixed feelings about the benefits that person-centred funding brings. Some feel there is nothing wrong with existing services, either because they want a 'safe haven' for their offspring, or because they do not realise there could be a different approach. Others have anxieties that their son or daughter's service will centre around the home and that they will get less of a break. Trail-blazing parents who have always wanted their children to have a more inclusive lifestyle are worried that this is something that, once again, they will have to fight for. Clements (1996) cautioned that Direct Payments may not empower people with severe learning difficulties, as it is often their parents who make all the decisions. He does, however, suggest that Direct Payments may be used to provide an improved service in terms of creating greater choice for daily living, but that this ultimately increases the financial and administrative burden on families.

To overcome these difficulties it is essential that the recommendations made within the White Paper regarding the dissemination of information are realised, so that people with learning disabilities, together with their families, are able to access information regarding what support is available at each stage of their lives.

Inter-agency working

Black (2000) comments that 'people in organisations often communicate poorly with one another' (p. 7). To address this enduring problem, the Department of Health has repeatedly emphasised the need for creating new partnership arrangements in order to promote a person-centred approach to the delivery of services. A starting point for many people will be the successful completion of Joint Investment Plans.

A service for all

Fruin (1998) reported that very few social services have a clear idea of the real unit costs involved in providing services. The Department of Health (1999) found that 'net expenditure is on an upward trend' (p. 24). Felce *et al.* (1998) have also commented on the cost of individualised support.

No matter how much money the Government proposes to spend on learning disability services it can never provide a seamless service. Even if the monies currently allocated to the maintenance of buildings-based services were used to fund individualised ones, some rationing would always exist. Many people with complex needs require one-to-one support sixteen hours a day or more, simply to address their health and personal care needs. Extra help will be required to enable them to participate in ordinary activities. Assessment of need is often used to apportion or ration the allocation of services. In a perfect world, a person with complex needs would be able to obtain as much help, paid or unpaid, as they desired. The reality of this is succinctly articulated by Dowson (1999) when he suggests that 'in the real world we cannot always have what we want: we often have to reconsider our aspirations as we find out what is possible' (p. 4). Although people with complex needs are unlikely to have any expectations of services, there will be a limit to the amount of assistance they will get. Inevitably the level of support will determine opportunities for inclusion.

The difficulties related to providing individual support was placed in context by a service manager, just after the publication of the White Paper. He reported that he was unable to release staff for training because he did not have enough people to run his day services. He said 'I have a year's waiting list for people who require one-to-one support. When I do find staff for them, I do it by removing support from other people.'

Conclusion

The title of this chapter posed the following question: is the inclusion of people with complex needs a reality or myth? The most important way to 'include' a person is to show that we value them by making certain that their physical and health care needs are sensitively and individually addressed. Sadly, many people are still denied this basic civil right. Additionally, many continue to endure a 'deprivation of contact and supportive networks' which has been clearly defined by the Department of Health (2001) No Secrets report as 'psychological abuse' (p. 9).

The notion of being included remains a myth, although it is apparent that when people with complex needs are listened to and their wants are clearly identified, their life improves (Sanderson 1998b; Routledge and Sanderson 2000). When the opposite occurs, they run the risk of being unhappy, isolated and abused. To try to examine whether people with complex needs are being included future service plans should at the very least consider how to:

- provide sensitive individualised personal *care*;
- provide *continuity* in a person's life;
- promote effective *communication*, with the individual concerned and all those who are involved in their life;
- promote a variety of interesting and *creative* models of support; and
- provide opportunities for transferring *control* from services to the individual.

Only when these issues are seriously addressed will people with complex needs truly start becoming participating members of everyday life.

References

Black, P. (2000) 'Why aren't person centred approaches and planning happening for as many people and as well as we would like'. Briefing paper. Joseph Rowntree, 29 November.

Bradley, H. (1998) Assessing and developing successful communication. In: P. Lacey and C. Ouvry (eds) *Profound and Multiple Learning Disabilities. A Collaborative Approach to Meeting Complex Needs*, London, David Fulton Publishers, pp. 50–65.

Caldwell, P. (1996) *Getting in Touch: Ways of Working with People with Severe Learning Disabilities and Extensive Support Needs*, Brighton, Pavilion Publishing.

Caldwell, P. and Stevens, P. (1998) *Person to Person: Establishing Contact and Communication with People with Profound Learning Disabilities and Extra Special Needs*, Brighton, Pavilion Publishing.

Cervi, B. (1996) Contracting rights. *Community Care*, 28 March–3 April: 22–23.

Clements, T. (1996) Direct Payments are they all good news? *Community Living* 10(2): 8–10.

Department of Health (1998a) *Moving into the Mainstream: The Report of a National Inspection of Services for Adults with Learning Disabilities*, London, The Stationery Office.

Department of Health (1998b) *Modernising Social Services: Promoting Independence; Improving Protection, Raising Standards*. Command Paper 4169, London, The Stationery Office.

Department of Health (1999) *Facing the Facts: Services for People with Learning Disabilities: Policy Impact Study of Social Care and Health Services*, London, The Stationery Office.

Department of Health (2000) *No Secrets: Guidance on Developing and Implementing Multi-agency Policies and Procedures to Protect Vulnerable Adults from Abuse*, London, The Stationery Office.

Department of Health (2001) *Valuing People. New Strategy for Learning Disability for the 21st Century*, London, The Stationery Office.

Dowson, S. (1998) *Certainties without Centres?*, London, Values into Action.

Dowson, S. (1999) *Who Does What? The Process of Enabling People with Learning Difficulties to Achieve What They Need and Want*, revised edition, London, Values Into Action.

Edge, J. (2001) *Who's in Control. Decision-making by People with Learning Difficulties Who have High Support Needs*, London, Values Into Action.

Emerson, E., Hatton, C, Robertson, J., Henderson, D. and Cooper, J. (1999) A descriptive analysis of the relationships between social context, engagement and stereotyping in residential services for people with severe and complex disabilities, *Journal of Applied Research in Intellectual Disabilities*, 12(1): 11–29.

Felce, D. (1999) The Gerry Simon Lecture, 1998: Enhancing the quality of life of people receiving residential support, *British Journal of Learning Disabilities*, 27: 4–9.

Felce, D. and Perry, J. (1995) Quality of life: its definition and measurement, *Research in Developmental Disabilities*, 16: 51–74.

Felce, D., Grant, G., Todd, S., Ramcharan, P., Beyer, S., McGrath, M., Perry, J., Shearn, J., Kilsby, M. and Lowe, K. (1998) *Towards a Full Life: Research on Policy Innovation for People with Learning Disabilities*, Oxford, Butterworth Heinemann.

Fruin, D. (1998) *Moving into the Mainstream: The Report of a National Inspection of Services for Adults with Learning Disabilities*, London, The Stationery Office.

Hatton, C. and Emerson, E. (1996) *Residential Provision for People with Learning Disabilities: A Research Review*, Manchester, Hester Adrian Research Centre.

Heller, T., Millar, A. and Factor, A. (1999) Adults with mental retardation as supports to their parents: effects on parental caregiving appraisal. *Mental Retardation*, 35(5): 338–346.

Holman, A. and Collins, J. (1998) Choice and control: Making direct payments work. In: L. Ward, *Innovations in Advocacy and Empowerment for People with Intellectual Disabilities*, Chorley, Lisieux Hall Publications, pp. 215–232.

Johnstone, D. (1998) *An Introduction to Disability Studies*, London, David Fulton Publishers.

King's Fund (1999) 'Learning disabilities: from care to citizenship', Briefing paper, June, London, King's Fund.

McIntosh, B. and Whittaker, A. (eds) (1998) *Days of Change*, London, King's Fund.

McIntosh, B. and Whittaker, A. (eds) (2000) *Unlocking the Future. Developing New Lifestyles with People Who have Complex Disabilities*, London, King's Fund Publishing.

Morris, J. (1999) *Hurtling into a Void. Transition to Adulthood for Young Disabled People with 'Complex Health and Support Needs'*, Brighton, Pavilion Publishing/Joseph Rowntree Foundation.

O'Brien, J. and Lyle O'Brien, C. (1996) *A Tune Beyond Us, Yet Ourselves. Power Sharing Between People with Substantial Disabilities and Their Assistants*, Lithonia, GA, Responsive Systems Associates.

O'Brien, J. and Lyle O'Brien, C. (2000) *The Origins of Person-Centred Planning. A Community of Practice Perspective*, Lithonia, GA, Responsive Systems Associates.

Poxton, P., Grieg, R. and Giraud Saunders, A. (2001) *Best Value Reviews of Learning Disability Services for Adults. A Framework for Applying Person Centred Principles*, London, The Stationery Office.

Rose, J. (1998) Measuring quality: the relationship between diaries and direct observations of staff, *British Journal of Developmental Disabilities* 44, 1(86): 30–36.

Routledge, M. and Sanderson, H. (2000) *Work in Progress. Implementing Person Centred Planning in Oldham*, Whalley, North West Training and Development Team.

Sanderson, H. (1998a) Person centred planning. In: P. Lacey and C. Ouvry (eds) *Profound and Multiple Learning Disabilities. A Collaborative Approach to Meeting Complex Needs*, London, David Fulton Publishers, pp. 130–145.

Sanderson, H. (1998b) A say in my future. Involving people with profound and multiple disabilities in person centred planning. In: L. Ward (ed.) *Innovations in Advocacy and Empowerment for People with Intellectual Disabilities*, Chorley, Lisieux Hall Publications, pp. 161–182.

Sanderson, H., Kennedy, J., Ritchie, P. and Goodwin, G. (1997) *People, Plans and Possibilities – Exploring Person Centred Planning*, Edinburgh, SHS.

Scottish Executive (2000) *The Same as You? A Review of Services for People with Learning Disabilities*, Scottish Executive.

Simons, K. (1999) *A Place at the Table?* Kidderminster, British Institute of Learning Disabilities Publications.

Simons, K. and Watson, D. (1999a) *The View from Arthur's Seat. A Literature Review of Housing and Support Options 'Beyond Scotland'*, Scottish Executive.

Simons, K. and Watson, D. (1999b) *New Directions? Day Services for People with Learning Disabilities in the 1990s*, Exeter Centre for Evidence-Based Social Services.

Smull, M. (1996) *Person Centred Planning, Should We do it to Everyone?* Support Development Associates. Online: http://www.allenshea.com/foreveryone.html (accessed 24/05/01).

Ward, C. (2000) *Family Matters. Counting Families In*, London, The Stationery Office.

Wertheimer, A. (ed.) (1996) *Changing Days: Developing New Day Opportunities with People Who have Learning Difficulties*, London, King's Fund.

Chapter 10

Advocacy and parents with learning difficulties

'Even when you've got an advocate Social Services still always do what's easiest for them'

Kathy Boxall, Michaela Jones and Shaun Smith

Introduction – how we wrote this chapter

Several years ago, Kathy acted as a short-term advocate for Shaun and Michaela and helped them make a complaint about the local Social Services Department. When Kathy contacted Shaun and Michaela recently and asked if they would be interested in writing this chapter with her, their response was an immediate 'yes' as they want as many people as possible to know about what happened to them and their family. Shaun and Michaela's names, the names of their children and other information which could identify them have all been changed.

When Kathy was Shaun and Michaela's advocate, we read some extracts from a book about parents with learning difficulties (Booth and Booth 1994). More recently, Kathy read some books and articles on her own and talked about what she had read with Shaun and Michaela. We agreed that Kathy would bring her tape recorder and record Shaun and Michaela talking about what they wanted to include in the chapter. We had four of these taped discussions, each lasting approximately forty-five minutes. We also had lots of telephone conversations and meetings which we didn't record on tape.

In one of our discussions Shaun stated bluntly:

> To be honest with you I think advocacy's crap. We've had a few advocates. They start, and then they stop when it's too complicated. The complaint was crap too, it didn't change anything.

Michaela added:

> Even when you've got an advocate, Social Services still always do what's easiest for them.

After each taped discussion, Kathy transcribed the tape. In the end, we found ourselves going round in circles and saying the same things over and over again.

Kathy reorganised some of what we had said on the tapes into a logical order. The bits where we went over the same things again were edited out.

Three years ago, Shaun and Michaela started writing their life stories. They asked for some help with this from the tutor of the literacy class they were attending but the tutor said they couldn't have any extra time. Two students from the learning difficulties degree course, Nicola and Michelle, volunteered to help them write their life stories. Shaun and Michaela would like to thank Nicola and Michelle for their help with this. We have included some of the information from the life stories in this chapter. We also used the notes that we made and the letters we wrote and received during the time when Kathy was Shaun and Michaela's advocate. Kathy put everything together and took it back to Shaun and Michaela so that that they could change anything she had written. We did this four times to make sure that everything was correct and there was nothing in the chapter that any of us were unhappy about. The final chapter is as agreed between the three of us.

We have written about our own experiences of advocacy. Ours is not a very positive story but we decided to write it because we feel it is important to record the limitations, frustrations and disappointments of advocacy rather than present a glossy picture. More optimistic accounts of citizen advocacy can be read in Paul Williams's (1998) collection of citizen advocacy stories.

During the course of our work for this chapter, Shaun and Michaela's circumstances changed and their priority became their present situation, rather than their past experiences of advocacy. Their contribution to the chapter therefore reflects these changed circumstances and their desired outcome that as many people as possible know about what happened (and continues to happen) to them.

We have divided the remainder of this chapter into five sections. These cover: forms of advocacy; citizen advocacy; our experience of citizen advocacy; self-advocacy; and Shaun and Michaela's current concerns.

Forms of advocacy

Wolf Wolfensberger (1977) notes that the term 'advocacy' only started appearing in human services literature around 1970. He points to a lack of familiarity with the concept at that time, to the extent that people even experienced difficulties with pronouncing the word 'advocacy'. Thirty years later, advocacy is a familiar term used without question by many service workers, students and people with learning difficulties. There appears to be an assumption that there's consensus about what advocacy is, and also that it is, of necessity, 'a good thing'. Closer examination, however, reveals differences of opinion about what counts as advocacy, and confusion about how, and by whom, it should be done (Atkinson 1999).

Wolfensberger points out that although the verb 'to advocate' means:

> to speak to a matter or issue. In time it has come to mean speaking on the behalf of a person or issue; and where a person is involved, it almost invariably has come to mean speaking on the behalf of *another* person, rather than oneself.
>
> (Wolfensberger 1977: 19)

There are several different forms of advocacy; lack of differentiation between these adds to confusion about what exactly is meant when the term 'advocacy' is used. Dorothy Atkinson's recent review provides a useful starting point when clarifying these different forms of advocacy.

> Advocacy takes many forms but is essentially about speaking up – wherever possible for oneself (self-advocacy), but sometimes with others (group or collective advocacy) and where necessary, through others. Speaking up 'through others' can involve another 'insider' (a peer advocate), an 'ordinary' person or volunteer (a citizen advocate), or a person trained and paid as an advocate (a paid advocate). All these types of advocacy are important in the health and social care fields. They co-exist but there are fundamental differences between them.
>
> (Atkinson 1999: 5)

In this chapter, we are going to look at two of these forms of advocacy: citizen advocacy and self-advocacy. We are going to start with citizen advocacy because that's how we first got to know each other – when Kathy became Shaun and Michaela's citizen advocate.

Citizen advocacy

Citizen advocacy has its origins in a 1966 conference in the USA where parents were expressing concern about what would happen to their sons and daughters with cerebral palsy when they died. Wolf Wolfensberger was present at the conference and came up with the idea of an unpaid citizen, unconnected with the services the person received, continuing to protect their interests when the family were no longer able to do so (Wertheimer 1998). Wolfensberger went on to develop the concept of citizen advocacy which he viewed as:

> a one-to-one relationship by which a competent citizen volunteer, free from built-in conflicts of interest, advances the welfare and interests of an impaired or limited person, as if that person's interests were the advocate's own.
>
> (Wolfensberger 1977: 31)

A citizen advocacy office, usually staffed by a co-ordinator, identifies a person in need of advocacy support. Wolfensberger refers to this person as the *protégé* (someone whose welfare is promoted by an influential person). In the UK, the term *partner* is usually used instead of *protégé*. The advocacy office recruits a citizen advocate specifically for that particular 'partner'. A profile of an ideal advocate with the skills and experience to meet the needs of the partner will have been drawn up by the co-ordinator and the advocate matched to that partner will have been chosen because they have the qualities which best meet their partner's needs. The citizen advocate and partner are introduced to each other by the advocacy co-ordinator who also provides ongoing support and advice to the advocate.

For Alison Wertheimer citizen advocacy's objectives are:

> to include those who have been excluded and to protect those who may need protection . . . Citizen Advocacy is a way of introducing people who probably would not otherwise meet. It invites ordinary members of the local community to meet and get to know vulnerable people, to understand their situation in life and to stand with them, one with one.
>
> (1998: 7)

In the late 1970s, John O'Brien and Wolf Wolfensberger developed *CAPE: Standards for Citizen Advocacy Program Evaluation* as a means of evaluating citizen advocacy (O'Brien and Wolfensberger 1988). CAPE sets out a series of citizen advocacy principles. The purpose of these principles is to minimise *conflict of interest*. Key principles may be summarised as follows:

- The citizen advocacy project should be independent from service providers.
- It should be managed by an independent management committee (none of whom work for services in the area).
- The advocacy office should proactively seek partners from diverse backgrounds, not rely on referrals.
- Citizen advocacy should be a one-to-one partnership.
- Citizen advocates should be valued citizens who are independent of services in the area.
- There should be no payment or compensation for advocates.
- The citizen advocate's primary loyalty should be to her/his partner, not to the co-ordinator or management committee.

The principles listed above are a simplified summary only. Readers should refer to O'Brien and Wolfensberger (1988) and Wertheimer (1998) for more comprehensive information.

Conflict of interest arises when there is a conflict between the interests of a particular partner and the interests of *someone* else (for example another partner) or *something* else (for example an organisation). The principles provide a possible means of achieving minimal conflict of interest: adherence to these principles should result in the interests of individual partners remaining paramount. Below, we describe an example from our own experience to help illustrate the concept of conflict of interest.

When Kathy was Shaun and Michaela's advocate she wrote a letter to the Director of Social Services stating that Shaun and Michaela were unhappy with the way their concerns had been dealt with and they wanted their complaint publicised. The letter was written on headed notepaper provided by the voluntary organisation which ran the advocacy project. This organisation was also a small-scale service provider and received some of its funding from Social Services. Although the advocacy project was separately funded by a lottery grant, the

Director of Social Services' response to Kathy's letter caused some concern within the voluntary organisation.

There are three potential areas of conflict of interest here.

First, Shaun and Michaela's complaint was about Social Services and Social Services provided some of the funding for the organisation which ran the advocacy project. The organisation was concerned to preserve its relationship with Social Services and asked to see any future letters Kathy wrote to the Social Services department. If anything she had written had been viewed contrary to the interests of the organisation, this would have placed the organisation's interests above those of Shaun and Michaela. In the event such conflict did not arise. However, the *potential* for conflict of interest remains. As stated above, citizen advocacy projects should be independent from service providers.

The second issue of conflict of interest concerns the advocate's primary loyalty: Kathy's primary loyalty should have been to Shaun and Michaela, not to what the advocacy co-ordinator or the voluntary organisation or indeed the Director of Social Services felt was in their best interests. She should have been free to do what she felt was in Shaun and Michaela's best interests.

The third issue concerns Kathy taking on the role of advocate for both Shaun and Michaela. On this occasion, they both wanted exactly the same outcome from their complaint to Social Services. However, had they wanted different outcomes, Kathy would have had to make a decision about who she was going to support. To minimise conflict of interest, the citizen advocacy relationship should be *one-to-one*: Shaun and Michaela should each have had their own advocate.

The citizen advocacy principles were developed in the USA. There has been debate among UK citizen advocacy projects as to the cultural appropriateness of the principles within the UK. There is some variation in the extent to which UK citizen advocacy projects adhere to the principles (see Simons 1993; Atkinson 1999). For example, the advocacy project with which we were associated reimburses advocates' out-of-pocket expenses, as do many other UK citizen advocacy projects. According to the principles, however, the advocate's time and any expense incurred should be freely given and not compensated (Wertheimer 1998).

Our experience of citizen advocacy

Kathy first met Shaun and Michaela in 1998 when they were making a complaint about their local Social Services department. Shaun and Michaela are disabled parents who have learning difficulties. They started going out with each other in 1985 and have lived together since 1987. They have two children, both of whom have been removed by Social Services. Shaun and Michaela's complaint was about the way the Social Services Department communicated with them when removing their children. A number of citizen advocates had already supported them in making this complaint but each one had left, either for personal reasons or because the complaints procedure had become too complex and difficult. At the point at which Kathy became involved, Shaun and Michaela's complaint had already been investigated by the local council under their Social Services' Complaints Procedure. This had involved a series of interviews by an independent investigator from a neighbouring Local Authority and had resulted in the complaint being upheld. A Social Services Review Panel followed. Shaun and Michaela remained unhappy about the outcome and decided to take the complaint to the Local Government Ombudsman. Kathy was asked by the local Advocacy Co-ordinator to act as a short-term advocate specifically in relation to Shaun and Michaela's communication with the Ombudsman.

Shaun and Michaela explain why they were unhappy about what Social Services did to their family and what happened when they made the complaint:

> Social Services took Becky, our second child, away soon after she was born and gave her up for adoption. Our six-year-old son Tony was also taken into care.
>
> Social Services had wanted Tony adopted when he was born. We had to go to court but the court ruled that Tony should live at home with us, with support from Social Services. When we found out that Michaela was pregnant with our second child we informed Social Services straight away. During the pregnancy, we had meetings with Social Services about the support we would need with the new baby. Then, without any consultation or warning, shortly before the birth, a letter was delivered to our house informing us that the new baby would be taken away and fostered at birth.
>
> We do agree with the law of the land, but Social Services should only remove a child as a last resort and if they have good reason to do so.
>
> We kept in contact with Social Services and we co-operated with them. They knew that we were having another baby. We told them about the things we were getting for the baby. They knew what we were doing but they didn't tell us until the last minute what they were going to do. They decided to post a letter through our door telling us that they wanted the baby fostering. They took the easy way out. They didn't think of us. It was done in a cruel and upsetting way for both of us. They should have thought about it much earlier in Michaela's pregnancy and told us what they wanted to do with Tony and Becky, then they would have had more time to find a family where Tony and Becky could have been together, which is what we would have wanted but only if Tony and Becky couldn't stay with us as a proper family.
>
> We've been discriminated against because we're disabled and have learning difficulties. We were already very traumatised by everything that Social Services did when Tony, our first child, was born. The same thing happened when Becky was born. It was like history repeating itself, only worse. We were very, very upset about what happened with Becky. We just got a letter through the door saying that they wanted Becky fostering. We weren't prepared. Our solicitor told us we would get Becky home but we didn't.
>
> We don't think that Social Services are all bad. We've had some good help from Social Services, a nursery place and help with bathing Tony, but we didn't get proper help with Tony's behaviour. We should have been given a

chance with Becky. We've seen programmes on TV where Social Services only take one of the children and help the parents with the other children. We don't know why Social Services took both of our children.

We still feel very upset about what happened. We think about it all the time. It's like bereavement, only it's worse than death because somebody else has got our children. Everything has been taken from under us in a very cruel and upsetting way. We don't want to have anything more to do with Social Services. We co-operated with them but they didn't co-operate with us. They stabbed us in the back instead. We can't just let this happen. We don't want the same thing to happen to anyone else, that's why we made the complaint.

We made a formal complaint to the Social Services Department about the way we were treated. Our complaint had three parts:

- the Social Services Department failed to provide adequate counselling and support up to the time our two children were removed;
- we were not told about the plan to remove our daughter at birth until near the time of the birth;
- we were told this by letter, not face to face.

Our complaint was upheld by an independent investigator. First of all we were offered £100 compensation for the money we had spent buying things for the new baby. We didn't accept the £100. Then we were offered £250 'as recompense for the expenditure we had incurred in purchasing items for the new baby and a recognition, albeit a very limited one, of the pain and distress we experienced'. We didn't accept this and Kathy helped us complain to the Local Government Ombudsman about the way Social Services had treated our family.

The Ombudsman wrote to us and asked what we thought Social Services should do to put things right. Kathy helped us write back. This is what we said:

- Disciplinary action should be taken against the person in Social Services who made the decision to post the letter through our door saying they wanted Becky fostered at birth. We don't want anyone else to be treated like we've been treated, that's why we feel that disciplinary action should be taken.
- Social Services should work in partnership with the families they work with and not adopt the attitude of 'we know best, your opinions don't count,' which is what happened to us when we became involved with the local Social Services team.
- There should be more training for staff around removing children from their parents and more information for parents in the early stages. We want to know what training Social Services staff have for working with disabled parents. What do the courses they go on tell them to do? Do they learn about the research that Wendy Booth has been doing in Sheffield?

- We also want adequate compensation from Social Services for the trauma, upset, stress and mental anguish caused to us by their maladministration and bad practice.

When the Ombudsman contacted Social Services about our complaint, Social Services just wrote back saying that they agreed that our complaint was justified, so the Ombudsman didn't bother to investigate our complaint anymore.

We didn't hear anything at all about what we'd said we'd like Social Services to do to put things right. The Ombudsman just told Social Services to increase the level of compensation they were offering to £500. We didn't accept the £500.

Michaela continues:

They shouldn't have done that. I mean, offering us £500 compensation; that was an insult. Five hundred pounds is nothing to us. It's like the next thing to death, what's happened to us. You know it's like a graveyard in here. It's not the same, just me and Shaun together, no Tony and Becky with us, I mean. It just feels lonely. If Social Services came to my door now, I'd just put the chain and the snip on and say 'Sorry, you're not coming in'. And I won't let them in. I won't have nothing to do with Social Services, never again. And that's a fact. And I think my Shaun feels the same about that too.

The stuff we bought for Becky, they didn't tell us 'til after. It was very disheartening for Shaun and me, selling all the stuff again. Them saying to us, 'Sorry, you can't keep Becky'. That puts all the stress on us. I mean they're being damn cruel. I'll never forget them what they did, never. I mean if I just see them walking around, I'll just ignore them. If they say 'Hello' to me I'll just ignore them, because I won't have nothing to do with them, ever again.

I think Social Services should have been answerable because they got away scot free, just taking the kids away from us for no reason at all, just because we're disabled. We can cope! There's people worse off than us having kids and their kids are brought home and we haven't got none of that. So where's our rights in that? We've got no rights at all. All we've gone through from what they've done.

If Shaun and I do go ahead with having another child, which we're hoping to do in the near future, we don't want nothing to do with Social Services whatsoever. We want them to back out.

Though their complaint had been upheld and the recommendation made that the compensation be increased to £500, Shaun and Michaela remained unhappy with the outcome and refused to accept the compensation. The process of writing to the Ombudsman and waiting for replies had also been extremely frustrating and disappointing for Shaun and Michaela.

The remit of complaints procedures, and therefore of complaints, is very narrow. Shaun and Michaela were unhappy about a number of aspects of their treatment by Social Services. Their deepest concern was the loss of their two children as a result of decisions made by the courts. These decisions were beyond the remit of either the Social Services' Complaints Procedure or the Ombudsman, as any complaints or challenges to legal decisions are deemed to lie within the legal system itself. Shaun and Michaela sought a Barrister's Opinion to see if they could qualify for Legal Aid to challenge these decisions but, because legal action on their behalf was considered unlikely to be successful, their application for Legal Aid was refused.

The Local Government Ombudsman's role is restricted to investigating 'maladministration' on the part of the Local Authority. Shaun and Michaela's primary motivation in pursuing the complaint had been to ensure that what had happened to them was in the 'public eye' and to improve things for future parents. The Social Services' Customer Relations Manager had assured Shaun and Michaela that the Ombudsman would publish their complaint. However, because the Ombudsman reached a settlement with the Local Authority, Shaun and Michaela's complaint, like 95 per cent of complaints to the Local Government Ombudsman, *was not formally investigated* (McDonald 1999). They received no reassurance that things would improve for other parents and their complaint was not publicised in any way. All three of us were left with the feeling that the whole business had been a time-consuming paper exercise that hadn't really changed anything at all. We hope that writing this chapter may at least help bring things out into the open.

Our experience of citizen advocacy also raises a number of other issues. Kathy was not Shaun and Michaela's advocate during the time when their two children were removed. It was some time after this that the local Advocacy Co-ordinator introduced us to each other. The three of us knew very little about the experiences of other parents with learning difficulties. Tim and Wendy Booth (1994) had carried out research in this area and we read about some of the families they had spoken to. We found that there were direct parallels between the experiences of these families and what happened to Shaun and Michaela's family.

Tim and Wendy Booth (1994) suggest that because of a 'presumption of incompetence' parents with learning difficulties are being treated more punitively than parents who do not have learning difficulties. David McConnell and Gwynnyth Llwellyn's (2000) research also found evidence of discrimination against parents with learning difficulties in statutory child protection proceedings across several different countries. They argue that throughout the process of child protection proceedings 'parents with intellectual disability are virtually powerless to challenge the evidence presented and to alter the likelihood that their children will be removed' (McConnell and Llwellyn 2000: 884).

Community care, as opposed to institutional care, is now a reality for many people with learning difficulties. Like other members of their communities, they may wish to participate fully in the rites and passages of family and community life. The Human Rights Act 1998, which came into force on 2 October 2000, incorporates into UK law *the protection of private and family life*. The extent to which the 'family life' of parents with learning difficulties will be protected remains to be seen. The Children Act 1989 is clear that it is the child's welfare that is paramount, not the needs or rights of the parents. On an individual level, it would appear that what is happening is that parents with learning difficulties are having their children removed because the child's needs can be better met elsewhere. However, as McConnell and Llwellyn (2000: 888) point out: there is also another explanation:

> The effect of focusing only on individual responsibility . . . spares the state the need to scrutinise its role in creating those difficulties. When the individual parent or their disability is viewed as the responsible agent, the 'problem' can be managed using the apparatus of the child protection system. An alternative focus on the larger societal context in which disability is constructed would force the child protection authorities to face an 'unmanageable' problem.

Within the UK there does appear to be at least some movement towards addressing this issue. *Valuing People* (DoH 2001) acknowledges the tensions and conflicts which may exist between the social workers whose focus is on the welfare of the child and other social services staff who are supporting the parents with learning difficulties. The White Paper states that, in addition to focusing on the needs of their children, future *child care* initiatives will also address the *needs of parents* with learning difficulties. The new 'Partnership Boards' are to be charged with responsibility for ensuring that services are in place to support parents with learning difficulties. Again, time will tell how this will translate into reality.

The White Paper also makes reference to advocacy, with promises of much-needed funding, and structures, for both citizen advocacy and self-advocacy. The definitions and descriptions of advocacy within the White Paper do not, however, reflect the tensions and complexities evident elsewhere. Dorothy Atkinson (1999: 25) writes of a 'tension at the heart of advocacy between citizen advocacy and the disability rights perspective'. Citizen advocacy involves a citizen advocate defending and advancing the welfare and interests of their partner as if that person's interests were the advocate's own. Wolfensberger (1977) is clear that citizen advocacy was intended for the people who need it the most; for example, people who don't speak or are 'profoundly impaired'. Where partners are unable to speak for themselves, there can be little disagreement about the benefit of having an advocate to speak on their behalf. If they are unable to assert their own interests, it may also be helpful for their advocate to defend their interests *as if they were the advocate's own*.

A problem arises with this model, however, when partners *are able to speak for themselves and wish to assert their own interests*, as was the situation when Kathy was Shaun and Michaela's advocate. Kathy sometimes had different ideas to Shaun and Michaela. Working to a pure citizen advocacy model, Kathy should have refused to support Shaun and Michaela in doing anything she felt wouldn't be in their best interests. This was very difficult. Kathy wanted Shaun and Michaela to have the same opportunities to control their own lives as other people, but she also recognised that we live in a very unequal society and wanted to protect Shaun and Michaela from some of the consequences of that unequal society.

Shaun and Michaela each have a lifetime's experience of being a disabled person with learning difficulties in our society. Kathy has no experience of this. Sometimes Kathy would think one thing was right but Shaun and Michaela would disagree. Shaun and Michaela would then talk about what had happened to them before. Sometimes Kathy would change her mind. Sometimes she wouldn't.

Within the disabled people's movement, disabled people are very clear about taking control of their own lives and have objected to the controlling influence of the medical profession.

> The control that we demand over our own lives is one that accepts that we are as irresponsible as everybody else and that we may not always do the right thing from a medical point of view. This is what I mean by the right to take risks. If we are to be treated as individuals who are due the same respect as other people, then we must be allowed to choose a way of living that confronts all the options and risks throughout life that are inherent to living in, rather than outside society.
>
> (Brisenden 1998 [1986]: 26)

Disabled people have also objected to relatives, social workers and other professionals controlling their lives (see, for example, Oliver 1990; Davis 1993). The idea of a citizen advocate who could also wrest control from disabled people in order to *act in their best interests* does not sit well with such objections. This is the tension with citizen advocacy. In our experience it has been a creative, if sometimes frustrating, tension which has led, among other things, to our jointly writing this chapter. Dorothy Atkinson's research, however, reveals less positive consequences.

> There is tension in the advocacy movement, sometimes overt conflict between its two main driving forces. This does not appear to be a creative tension, instead it seems to be a divisive process. Projects are run in parallel, seeking separate funding and separate human resources; creating a competitive, rather than a collaborative environment.
>
> (Atkinson 1999: 26)

Dorothy Atkinson's research also found citizen advocates taking on tasks which would more usually be undertaken by social workers and her report concludes by suggesting that advocacy has the potential to become 'an informal community-based branch of social work' (Atkinson 1999: 42). This is something which concerns us. In our view, the tension between citizen advocacy and the disability rights perspective has had a positive effect on citizen advocacy. Without it, we feel there would be a *risk* that citizen advocacy could become just like social work.

In relation to people with learning difficulties, 'the disability rights perspective' has more usually been referred to as *self-advocacy* – people 'sticking up for themselves' or speaking on their own behalf. We believe that self-advocacy and citizen advocacy should go hand in hand, which is what we tried to do when Kathy was helping Shaun and Michaela make their complaint about Social Services.

Self-advocacy

Dan Goodley (2000: 7) points out that 'literature on self-advocacy has tended to focus on the doing of self-advocacy in the formal context of groups'. He cites a range of literature sources which trace the origins of the self-advocacy movement to the 1960s. Conferences were organised in Sweden and the USA which brought together large groups of people with learning difficulties who spoke up about the changes they would like to see happen in services. In the UK, The Campaign for the Mentally Handicapped (CMH) organised similar conferences or 'Participation Events' in the early 1970s. More recently, self-advocacy has taken place within smaller groups where people with learning difficulties meet together and speak out about issues which concern them in order to try and bring about change. Some of these groups are located within services for people with learning difficulties. Other groups, in order to avoid conflict of interest, are independent of services. Some self-advocacy groups, both inside and outside services, go under the name of 'People First' and are part of a wider, international movement of self-advocacy groups. A number of national and international People First conferences have been held in recent years (Aspis 1997; Bersani 1998; Goodley 2000; Dowse 2001).

Self-advocacy is ostensibly about people with learning difficulties taking control of their own lives. However, as Simone Aspis (1997) points out, the self-advocacy of people with learning difficulties is, in the main, under the control of service providers. Even the name *self-advocacy* is something which has been dreamt up by the service system to describe what people with learning difficulties are doing when they complain about services (Dowson 1990).

Simone Aspis describes herself as 'a disabled person who has been labelled by the system as having learning difficulties' (1999: 174). In an article about the future of self-advocacy, she explains that throughout their lives people with learning difficulties have been socialised into depending upon service providers for positive attention or approval in order to feel valued. In her experience, the self-advocacy training that services offer people with learning difficulties focuses on interpersonal and communication skills and does not examine legal rights or power relationships. She argues that self-advocacy groups based within services are being used to find out what people with learning difficulties think of services. Even the 'independent' self-advocacy groups are being contracted by services to provide 'user expertise'. This, combined with the dependency-inducing power relationships between service providers and people with learning difficulties 'means that service providers . . . are dictating what people with learning difficulties should be speaking up about' (Aspis 1997: 652).

Dan Goodley offers a more favourable description of self-advocacy:

> Self-advocacy can be seen as a counter-movement to state paternalism, wherein people with the label of learning difficulties conspicuously support one another to speak out against some of the most appalling examples of discrimination in contemporary British culture. The self-advocacy movement has invited people with learning difficulties to revolt against disablement in a variety of ways, in a number of contexts, individually and collectively, with and without the support of others. The movement captures resilience in the face of adversity.
>
> (Goodley 2000: 3)

We agree that people with learning difficulties are speaking out about their experiences and are doing this with strength and conviction. But the self-advocacy that many people with learning difficulties are being sold amounts to an abbreviated version of the political force of the disabled people's movement. In recent years, Shaun and Michaela have watched numerous television programmes featuring disabled activists and their organisations. They too would like to be part of this movement. Shaun wants to organise a rally for disabled parents who have had their children removed by Social Services. He has not had any success in getting this off the ground. When he and Michaela approached the local organisation of disabled people, the response they received was 'Sorry, but we can't help you'.

This echoes Simone Aspis's experience of the disability movement:

> People with learning difficulties face discrimination in the disability movement. People *without* learning difficulties use the medical model when dealing with us.
>
> (Simone Aspis, in Campbell and Oliver 1996: 97, emphasis added)

Leanne Dowse (2001: 134) argues that people with learning difficulties' *restricted* collective experience of oppression has contributed to their marginalisation within the disabled people's movement. She suggests that some people with learning difficulties have 'cognitive limitations' which mean that their collective experience of oppression may be limited to 'self advocacy in service based speaking up groups'. Because of this, she argues, they may be unable to identify with the oppression of other disabled people. This view firmly locates the 'problem' within the individual with learning difficulties and serves to illustrate Simone Aspis's comment above. It also belies the collective experience of people with learning difficulties outwith formalised advocacy settings. Many people's experiences of institutional and segregated services were (and still are) *collective* experiences of oppression. Maggie Potts and Rebecca Fido (1991) record the memories of former residents of 'The Park' colony, who articulated concerns about the unfair treatment meted out to other patients, as well as themselves:

There were some nasty nurses what used to work there. We're only human, but they were cruel (Grace).

(109)

We weren't able to mix with any of the female patients . . . We were never told the reason for it. I didn't see any reason for it at all. I just didn't see any reason for it (Ernest).

(111)

When David Barron (1996) writes about the injustices he experienced within Whixley Institution, he also expresses concern for the harsh, unfair treatment that other patients received.

Another possible factor in the development of collective identity is the broadcasting of television programmes which look at disability issues. Television is a medium which is immediately accessible to many people with learning difficulties. Some people with learning difficulties who watch disability programmes will, like Shaun and Michaela, identify with the experiences of the disabled people *without* learning difficulties they see in these programmes.

Shaun and Michaela are clear that they want to participate *fully* in the disabled people's movement. They want to both contribute to, and share, the collective power of its membership.

All three of us feel that without the political power of the wider disabled people's movement, there is a risk that self-advocacy will become, as Simone Aspis has argued, 'a tool to support people with learning difficulties to accept the best out of a bad deal' (1997: 653). We also have similar concerns about citizen advocacy, particularly in relation to parents with learning difficulties. When Kathy was Shaun and Michaela's advocate, she felt as if she had been 'sent in' to persuade Shaun and Michaela to 'accept the best out of an *appallingly* bad deal'.

While we are encouraged by the model of advocacy support for parents with learning difficulties which Wendy and Tim Booth (1998) describe, Shaun and Michaela are only too aware of the discrimination and powerlessness which parents with learning difficulties face within the child protection system. With or without advocacy support, we do not feel optimistic about Shaun and Michaela's current concerns.

Shaun and Michaela's current concerns

During the time we've been writing this chapter, Shaun and Michaela's circumstances have changed. They have recently discovered that Michaela is pregnant again. They want their current concerns to be in the 'public eye'.

Michaela continues:

When I have my third child, I expect to keep my third child with Shaun and me because Shaun and me really love each other and we'd like to be together as a family, the three of us: me, Shaun and the baby. Wherever we go, we'll always have the baby home. And I don't want it to happen like it happened with Tony and Becky being took away. I want to keep the baby. I don't want the same thing to happen again, that's why I don't want to go to court. But I know it is going to go to court. If I can keep the baby for more than two or three years there'll be more chance they won't take it from me as long as I'm looking after it well.

Shaun and I just want to settle down and get on with our own lives. With me, Shaun and the baby. When we had Tony we did the feeding ourselves and the changing and that, but the only one problem we had was bathing Tony. I could manage to bath the new baby myself, if I had help. I couldn't manage doing all by myself, but with help I could do it, if someone taught me what to do slowly and carefully. Babies need a lot of love. Caring and cuddling, loving from the both of us. I tried breast-feeding with Tony and then I found it a bit uncomfortable then I bottle fed and I was alright with that. We can change nappies, disposable nappies, not towelling ones. Both of us can do it on our own.

I know my Shaun will support me; he'll support me every step of the way in having our child. I'm getting these kicking pains in me tum and real backache at night and I sometimes get a bit uncomfortable watching telly so I stick about three or four cushions behind me back. We feel proud when we feel the baby kicking. Shaun's over the moon.

Shaun continues:

I want to save the happiness to when the baby's born. We're very pleased we're having the baby, but we've got a lot of work to do because we want to get this baby home.

Social Services don't know yet that we're expecting this baby. We've seen our real GP once; she said she can't make a comment on it but she sympathises with us. The first time we went to the doctor we saw a temporary GP. The temporary GP didn't want to refer Michaela to St Angela's Hospital, she just wanted us to go back to the same hospital as last time but we wouldn't agree to that. When we got to St Angela's, we found out that the temporary GP had written a letter to the hospital. It said 'This couple have had two children before. Both children were removed by Social Services. They're not capable of bringing up the new baby and the baby's got rights.' That offended us. The midwife was shocked by the letter too. She told us about it and she's spoken to the Advocacy Co-ordinator about it as well.

We'll have to go to court in the end. People like us always have to go to court when they have a baby. You know that, I know that. Wendy Booth's book says that.

I must stress out. There's no way I'm going to be blackmailed by the State. They could say 'If you want to keep the baby you're going to have to work with Social Services'. Why should I work with Social Services? I've worked with them for the last ten years and they just scarred me and we got trod on. All they was doing was looking at the baby – they weren't interested in us. But there again, I want people to help me and Michaela look after the baby, so we can be together as a family unit. We'd like help with the baby, not Social Services watching us in a fishbowl, waiting for us to do something wrong. There's too much damage been done with our relationship with Social Services. We'd like help from another organisation, not Social Services.

The most important thing is to keep the baby.

What I'm jealous of is that a few weeks ago, this murderer, he took his case to the House of Lords. He got to the House of Lords, but I can't get to the House of Lords can I? I'm still stuck here. I should be entitled to the highest court in the land. I haven't done anything wrong. But I can't budge anymore can I? The whole system's against me. I'm powerless against the law of the land. Becky shouldn't have been put up for adoption but she went for adoption didn't she? I think that's wrong. You do everything by the book and you still can't get anywhere.

We don't want no more assessments. We know we have to look after the baby. We will. We know what to do:

Love the baby.
Be honest about what things we can't do with the baby, so it's not a failure.
Don't do anything to upset the baby.
Don't neglect the baby.
Do our best with the baby. No one's perfect.

Everyone makes mistakes. I made mistakes with Tony. I smacked him when I lost my temper with him. I told Social Services. I asked Social Services for help with disciplining Tony and they wouldn't help. I wasn't advised what to do, what sort of emotions he was going through. We didn't know why he was doing things like throwing eggs at the window and no one was helping us to find out why he was doing it. I've been watching programmes on TV where families go away and have help with the children's behaviour, learning how to control it and have tests for food allergies and things like that. They get the children back to their proper behaviour and they're allowed to stay living at home with their parents. It's not only us that's had problems with our children's behaviour, other people get help, but we weren't given that chance.

We've got a new solicitor now and she says we can have a pre-birth assessment for the new baby. She also said that when the baby's born it should stay in hospital as long as possible, but for us that's very stressful. It's very stuffy and hot and humid and you see people coming in and having their babies and then going home with their babies. And all the time you've got to be thinking about what Social Services are up to and that, what they're trying to do to you, to get the baby fostered out. The baby should stay in hospital if there's something wrong with it or feeding problems, not if there's nothing wrong with it.

A newborn baby's very vulnerable isn't it? It can easily be sucked out of your hands by Social Services, even if you're not doing anything wrong.

Even if we're looking after it properly, they can still do that can't they?

References

Aspis, S. (1997) Self-advocacy for people with learning difficulties; does it have a future?, *Disability & Society*, 12(4): 647–654.

Aspis, S. (1999) What they don't tell disabled people with learning difficulties. In: M. Corker and S. French (eds) *Disability Discourse*, Buckingham, Open University Press.

Atkinson, D. (1999) *Advocacy: A Review*, York, Joseph Rowntree Foundation.

Barron, D. (1996) *A Price to be Born: My Childhood and Life in a Mental Institution*, Harrogate, Mencap Northern Division.

Bersani, H. (1998) From social clubs to social movement: landmarks in the development of the international self-advocacy movement. In L. Ward (ed) *Innovations in Advocacy and Empowerment for People with Intellectual Disabilities*, Chorley, Lisieux Hall Publications.

Booth, T. and Booth, W. (1994) *Parenting under Pressure: Mothers and Fathers with Learning Difficulties*, Buckingham, Open University Press.

Booth, W. and Booth, T. (1998) *Advocacy for Parents with Learning Difficulties: Developing Advocacy Support*, Brighton, Pavilion Publishing.

Brisenden, S. (1998 [1986]) Independent living and the medical model of disability. In: T. Shakespeare (ed.) *The Disability Reader: Social Science Perspectives*, London, Cassell, pp. 20–27.

Campbell, J. and Oliver, M. (1996) *Disability Politics: Understanding Our Past, Changing Our Future*, London, Routledge.

Davis, K. (1993) The crafting of good clients. In: J. Swain, V. Finkelstein, S. French and M. Oliver (eds) *Disabling Barriers – Enabling Environments*, London, Sage.

Department of Health (2001) *Valuing People: A New Strategy for Learning Disability for the 21st Century*, London, The Stationery Office.

Dowse, L. (2001) Contesting practices, challenging codes: self advocacy, disability politics and the social model, *Disability & Society*, 16(1): 123–141.

Dowson, S. (1990) *Keeping It Safe: Self-advocacy by People with Learning Difficulties and the Professional Response*, London, Values Into Action.

Goodley, D. (2000) *Self-advocacy in the Lives of People with Learning Difficulties*, Buckingham, Open University Press.

McConnell, D. and Llwellyn, G. (2000) Disability and discrimination in statutory child protection proceedings, *Disability & Society*, 15(6): 883–895.

McDonald, M. (1999) *Understanding Community Care: A Guide for Social Workers*, Basingstoke, Macmillan.

O'Brien, J. and Wolfensberger, W. (1988) *CAPE: Standards for Citizen Advocacy Program*

Evaluation, Syracuse, Training Institute for Human Service Planning, Leadership & Change Agentry.

Oliver, M. (1990) *The Politics of Disablement*, Basingstoke, Macmillan.

Potts, M. and Fido, R. (1991) *'A Fit Person to Be Removed': Personal Accounts of Life in a Mental Deficiency Institution*, Plymouth, Northcote House.

Simons, K. (1993) *Citizen Advocacy: The Inside View*, Bristol, Norah Fry Research Centre.

Wertheimer, A. (1998) *Citizen Advocacy: A Powerful Partnership*, London, Citizen Advocacy Information and Training.

Williams, P. (1998) *Standing by Me: Stories of Citizen Advocacy*, London, Citizen Advocacy Information and Training.

Wolfensberger, W. (1977) *A Multi-component Advocacy/Protection Schema*, Toronto, Canadian Association for the Mentally Retarded.

Part IV

Academia and learning disability – two debates

Chapter 11

The 'normalisation' debate – time to move on

David Race

Introduction

When the course at Stockport College moved from a Diploma to a full degree in Professional Studies (Learning Difficulties) in 1992 'normalisation' would have been a subject that any such course would make mandatory, given the influence of the set of ideas under this heading in the late 1970s and 1980s, an influence acknowledged by supporters, critics and neutral observers alike (Brown and Smith 1992). At the same time, however, the early 1990s saw a rapid growth in academic critics of 'normalisation', especially in the UK, and the parallel development of what became seen as an alternative, or even a replacement, namely the social theory of disability (see Kathy Boxall's discussion in Chapter 12). Meanwhile, the progress of 'Social Role Valorization' (SRV), Wolfensberger's reformulation and development of his version of 'normalization' into what he described, in the title of his last published monograph to date (1998), as 'a high order concept for addressing the plight of societally devalued people, and for structuring human services', was taking place in North America, Australasia, Norway, and, to a much smaller extent, in the UK.

As a result of this strange mixture – of perceived power over services of 'normalisation'; of reaction from the service world as the mere placing of people in community settings proved insufficient to deal with the devaluation that the ideas had highlighted; and of academic attacks which ranged from serious debate to hysterical, ill-informed and personalised vitriol; the possibility of SRV being considered seriously and intellectually became virtually nil. In particular the inability of what Tyne (1994) described as three 'movements' – normalisation, advocacy and the self-organisation of disabled people – to form alliances against devaluation left the still dominant system, the medical model, with a ragged and bickering opposition. While some of the roots of the policies now put forward in the 2001 White Paper can be 'claimed' by one or other of the three 'movements', the place and influence of SRV in those policies is implicitly, if not explicitly, denied. If, however, we examine the objectives of the White Paper against the primary and secondary goals of SRV, as we shall do later, the concordance is striking.

The medium and the messengers – fact and fiction in the communication of ideas into practice

For something that had an approximately eight hundred item bibliography published in 1999 (Flynn and Lemay) and has been around in one form or another for over thirty years, one might expect that some clarity would exist as to the development and implementation of ideas and theories from the root called normalisation. An examination of many of the references in that bibliography that emanate from the UK, however, would suggest, if taken at face value, the following: that the phenomenon of 'normalisation' subsumes both SRV and the 'Five Service Accomplishments' put forward by O'Brien (1987); and that all three are subject to the same criticisms of being service controlled, associated with a person in Wolfensberger whose views on other issues make even listening to his theory 'unacceptable' and which, by the very naming and analysis of devaluation, contribute to the oppression of vulnerable people (Ramcharan *et al.* 1997).

Very few of those UK references cite accounts of the development of normalisation from people who were actually there. In 1994, two such people, Wolf Wolfensberger and Bengt Nirje, explained to the first international SRV conference in Ottawa just how fragile, in both Europe and North America in the 1960s and early 1970s, were the chances of anything like normalisation being implemented (Flynn and Lemay 1999, chapters 2 and 3). From those accounts, too, the particular position of the UK, through the association with Tizard, also gives some clues as to why this country initially took up a particularly institutional and medically oriented view of normalisation. Again, this is covered in detail elsewhere (Race 1999a, 1999b), with particular reference to the contemporary criticisms of Shearer, one of the founder members of CMH (see Chapter 2). It took another member of CMH, Alan Tyne, together with Paul Williams, to use the developments of training that had already been widespread in the USA and Canada, via workshops based on the PASS instrument (Wolfensberger and Glenn 1975), to really bring normalisation in practice to this country.

The details of those developments are, like much of the 'normalisation' story, surrounded more by myths than realities, and only two elements are selected here. The first concerns the main medium used for this development, and the second concerns the parts played by the principal overseas contributors, John O'Brien and Wolf Wolfensberger. Both have told their own stories elsewhere (Wolfensberger 1999a, 1999b; Lyle O'Brien and O'Brien 2000), though in an international context, so readers may like to see how this partial and personal account differs or agrees with theirs. It is written with great respect to their respective contributions.

The medium – CMHERA and PASS and PASSING workshops

To return to the first point, however, it is my contention that the rise of normalisation in the UK would not have occurred in as powerful a way had the medium of the PASS workshop not been used by Tyne and Williams, via their training organisation, spun off from CMH, called the Community and Mental Handicap Education and Research Association (CMHERA). It is also, however, my contention that the service and academic backlash, and the weak development of SRV as a distinct theory in the UK, had its roots in that same medium of the PASS workshop. Both contentions say much about the particular nature of UK services and academia, especially in the perceived backwater of a subject that is learning disability.

PASS (and later PASSING, Wolfensberger and Thomas 1983) workshops had been developed in the 1970s in North America, especially by a group of people working with Wolfensberger at the National Institute for Mental Retardation (now the Roehrer Institute) in Toronto. They are intensive events, involving long hours of analysis and discussion of real services and their effects on real people (see Chapter 7). Above all, they provide a profound insight into the effects of devaluation on people's lives, and of the contribution of services to this. The fact that these insights are afforded to people from all levels of services, and also non-service people such as relatives and carers, made PASS(ING) workshops a powerful tool to influence services. What they are less good at doing *on their own*, in my view, is teaching the theory, both of normalisation but even more so of SRV, which was being first formulated just as PASSING came out in 1983.

Whether that matters then depends on one's view of the importance of ideas being fully understood to be effective, or theories being fully developed and criticised before being put into effect. As I will try to explain later in this chapter, I believe the foundation of normalisation, as of SRV, is an understanding, *at both a conceptual and emotional level*, of the power and effects of devaluation, on individuals, groups, and whole sections of society. The effects of PASS and PASSING workshops were, on the whole, very successful on the latter front, which to me explains their power with grass roots and first-line service workers. They were less successful, though by no means absolutely so, at the conceptual level. This, I suggest, is partly due to the intellectually hierarchical way in which services and academia have been structured in the UK, so that those at the top tend to look somewhat askance at teaching which demands they get their hands dirty, both with service users and front-line staff. It also, ironically, feeds off the reverse of that phenomenon, also common in my experience of academia and human services, where an attitude of suspicion and even hostility is displayed towards any ideas that demand detailed intellectual engagement. This has been especially powerful in the reaction to normalisation of those seeking to promote self-determination and the rights of people with learning difficulties, where the language of PASS and PASSING, as well as Wolfensberger's reformulation of SRV, has been described as 'elitist' or 'jargon' (e.g. Ramcharan *et al.* 1997).

The particular development of PASS and PASSING workshops in the UK has, I believe, added to that double-edged sword. PASS workshops in the UK were based on the US model, but in the form developed and practised by John O'Brien and others (O'Brien 1985), which CMHERA, in particular Paul Williams with PASSING workshops, then refined further. There are a number of technical issues here of which space precludes discussion, but the main difference, from my perspective, was the inclusion, in one and the same workshop, of theory presentations and the practical analysis of real services. What this tended to result in (and I speak from personal experience of having done exactly this) was a dilution of the theoretical presentation content to allow sufficient space for the practical work. O'Brien's style, based around 'story-telling' and evocative insights stemming from individual stories, was taken up by CMHERA presenters, often with equal quality and equal impact to the charismatic O'Brien. This, however, increasingly diverged from the methods used by Wolfensberger's Training Institute and others who followed their leadership process, where three- and four-day 'theory events' became separate from, and a prerequisite for, PASS and PASSING workshops. The divergence was compounded by Wolfensberger's development, especially by the early 1990s, of SRV as a theoretical concept distinct from normalisation, and the abandonment, in the circles that looked to him for guidance, of PASS as a teaching tool in favour of PASSING. So one edge of the sword cut into the ability of those in the UK to discuss and communicate SRV as a set of conceptual ideas, though again reaction to this depends on the importance placed on conceptual ideas as being influential.

The other edge, meanwhile, was honed by the academic criticisms of 'normalisation' (with 'Social Role Valorisation' sometimes being used interchangeably). Initially, academics had been noticeably quiet on normalisation, at least in terms of discussing the ideas theoretically. The move to SRV therefore had no real base of debate to set itself against. Even Wolfensberger (1998: 1) himself states, 'the early article-length overviews of SRV [Wolfensberger 1983, 1984, 1985] were much too short to give an adequate grasp of SRV'. Very little literature, either on normalisation or, certainly, on SRV, had appeared in mainstream UK textbooks or journals in the early 1980s. Then, in 1985, Wolfensberger made the first of a number of visits to the UK, of which more in the next section, speaking to audiences largely from the growing 'movement' developed by CMHERA and their network. The fact that he spoke about other issues than SRV, putting forward some controversial views, combined with the confusion about normalisation, seems to have been strongly reflected in the academic literature of the late 1980s and early 1990s. Academics could not deny the impact of normalisation, via CMHERA's influence in particular, on services. Yet they could not, or did not, with a few exceptions (e.g. Alaszewski and Ong 1990) discuss the ideas themselves and particularly the notion of SRV as a significant development from normalisation, since they had little UK or any other literature to work with.

As noted above, therefore, though 'SRV-specific' teaching grew elsewhere in the world especially Australasia, in the early 1990s, (Millier 1999), the contemporary development by Wolfensberger of SRV into a full-blown social science theory, which emerged formally at the 1994 Ottawa conference, went largely unnoticed in the UK training world, and even less in the academic world. By then, the effects of other pressures, particularly those discussed in Chapter 6, had transformed the service world and the academic world to such a position that it was difficult to imagine any one set of ideas having such an impact again. In addition, the relative views on the two overseas 'messengers' had by then taken on such force in the UK that anything coming from Wolf Wolfensberger was treated with deep suspicion, while John O'Brien, very often without his knowing anything about it, was having his ideas used and abused much as normalisation had been in the previous decade.

The messengers – John O'Brien and Wolf Wolfensberger

The separation, for the purposes of this chapter, into the 'medium and the messengers' is of course merely a device of my own to try and tease out the experiences of 'normalisation' and SRV in the UK. It is not my intention to deny either the quality or quantity of the work of large numbers of people in this country attempting to grapple with and put over the ideas, nor to reopen personality and power issues that have been long gone, if not forgotten. The point is to look at why SRV theory has never really been widely discussed in the UK merely on its own merits, as an interesting concept that may still have some relevance to the development of services and responses to the devaluation of vulnerable groups. Some of this has to do with these two messengers, who once worked together, have now gone in different directions, each with their own 'followers' (though I suspect they would both dislike the term and the phenomenon), and who, I believe, both sincerely want to get good things happening for vulnerable people.

We have seen how CMHERA developed workshops very much reflecting the style of O'Brien and what he refers to as the 'community of practice' that had tried to implement initiatives from the common experiences of teaching about normalisation through PASS (Lyle O'Brien and O'Brien 2000). In addition to being involved with PASS workshops, and as an extension of attempts at change that resulted from them, O'Brien has been, from the 1980s onwards, a regular visitor to the UK in consultancy and training roles. These attempts at change, often with CMHERA but also with a growing network of others, were concerned with the implementation of strategies to progress beyond the identification of the problem of devaluation that normalisation and PASS provided. Many of the service developments that were held up as models of 'values in practice' (e.g. Harper 1990) had a significant input from him. He was also involved: in the developing Citizen Advocacy movement, another idea from Wolfensberger that grew and was implemented very differently in the UK than elsewhere; in work with people with learning difficulties themselves, in various forms including self-advocacy; and in developments of the ideas that became subsumed under the heading of 'inclusion', especially in education.

As he explains in his paper at the Ottawa conference (O'Brien, in Flynn and Lemay 1999) most of this work involves attempting to develop what he describes as the 'practical arts of improving services for people with disabilities'. That paper describes a 'crossroads' for people who had worked on normalisation (including, of course, those in the UK) coming when the full implications of devaluation were realised. One path to take, which he himself had chosen, was to try and 'climb up the path of creation'. This involves many aspects and efforts, not least involvement with disabled people, an awareness of the multi-dimensional nature of change, and 'articulation of a vision or image of a desirable future'. At the second International SRV Conference in 1999 (as yet unpublished) O'Brien used an analogy of the 'swamps of practice' as opposed to the 'trees of theory', with his own twist on the notion of himself as a 'dinosaur' for continuing to talk about normalisation and PASS. The point I think he was making was that it is important for at least some people to respond to devaluation by trying to devise ways of making small amounts of progress whilst still acknowledging devaluation's strength and pervasiveness.

Going back to his impact on the UK, then, one such approach was a workshop called 'Framework for Accomplishment' (O'Brien and O'Brien 1989). This was promoted in the UK by CMHERA, especially Alan Tyne, in the late 1980s and from it came a set of themes, around which services might develop their 'accomplishments' in helping people, their families and communities, in becoming 'members one of another'. Ironically, however, the list of 'Five Accomplishments' gave the movement and the services, as well as a very useful developmental tool, a much less painful analysis than PASS(ING), and the sort of language that can be much more readily put into service planning documents and statements of vision. The fact that O'Brien has made clear several times the distinction between normalisation and his formulation of accomplishments (O'Brien and O'Brien 1989; O'Brien 1999; Lyle O'Brien and O'Brien 2000) has not prevented a widespread acceptance in the UK of his ideas as being an 'alternative version' of normalisation (e.g. Emerson 1992) with, in one textbook widely used in nurse training, Gates (1997), the claim that O'Brien and Tyne wrote them in their 1981 CMH pamphlet on normalisation. Though the workshops ceased being taught by the mid-1990s, 'knowledge of', and often 'adherence to' O'Brien's 'Five Accomplishments' became commonplace as requirements in job descriptions. So O'Brien's place, as a teacher, consultant and teller of 'good news', was, and is, firmly established in the learning disability world in this country, and many still also regard him as the embodiment of normalisation, (or, even more confusingly, SRV), whatever he may say to the contrary, and however many other important things, such as advocacy, inclusion and person-centred planning he may become involved with.

For Wolfensberger, the UK was to become a much less welcoming place, and with it the interest in SRV as he was developing it. Though the divergence over training discussed above might not have been that apparent to those outside the small number of people closely involved, we have noted another dimension that arose in the late 1980s and into the 1990s which was to cause yet more dissension and confusion, both within the narrow circle of the 'movement' and in the wider service and academic world, and which continues to this day. This dimension was the series of visits to the UK, from the mid-1980s onwards and to initially large audiences, of Wolfensberger himself, usually with his associate Susan Thomas.

Because of the power of the 'social movement', even by 1985 when he first came, and certainly by the later visits towards the end of the 1980s, very many people were interested in listening to Wolfensberger's presentations. The problem, however, of those visits, as far as the development of SRV was concerned, was that the presentations did not deal much with SRV, but instead focused on Wolfensberger's wider, some would say higher level, concerns. These included, among other things, the changing values of western society, the growth of what he termed the Post Primary Production Economy, and the massive increase, as he saw it, in the threat to the lives of vulnerable people. Though these views were published variously (Wolfensberger 1989a, 1989b), the real impact on the 'social movement' came from the actual presentations themselves.

First, the style was similar to the Training Institute style for SRV theory events, with extensive lecture presentations and use of multiple overhead projectors. This, as we have seen, was unfamiliar to the UK training scene, especially in the predominantly social work and psychology world from which his audience came, even those who were involved in normalisation. More importantly, the views presented, especially on 'deathmaking', as far as many feminists were concerned, and on higher-order issues of beliefs, as far as agnostic, atheist or other religious sceptics were concerned, a major challenge to the values of his audiences, both those in the 'network' and those academics receiving second-hand accounts of the events. To those on the edges of the 'social movement' it often appeared that they were being asked to take Wolfensberger 'all or nothing', though he made strenuous efforts to separate out the developing theory of SRV from his other views. To those academics, however, looking for ways to attack the power of normalisation, the 'political incorrectness' of some of Wolfensberger's views provided the perfect argument, decidedly *ad hominem*.

Further, from within the 'movement' in the late 1980s, there appeared to some to be two 'orthodoxies' developing: on SRV from Wolfensberger and his Training Institute, and, in the UK, on normalisation from CMHERA. Those seeking to be 'more like' Wolfensberger's Training Institute in their presentation of SRV saw CMHERA as 'holding on' to their way of doing things, i.e. the O'Brien way. On the other hand those seeking to develop and broaden training methods around the general ideas (including CMHERA with the 'Framework' workshops and others) saw the 'leadership ladder' of the Training Institute as a de facto control over what and how they could teach.

So despite the lack of progress in developing the brave new 'post-normalisation' world, especially for people with learning difficulties, and despite the maintenance and development of the applicability of SRV in other countries and for other vulnerable groups, the theory is little studied, let alone taught, in the UK. Some have attempted to make some inroads on that in the academic world (Race 1999a). Others have attempted to bring in SRV training as part of an overall service development, or for other vulnerable groups, but still it remains tarred with its own history. In the remainder of this chapter, therefore, I will attempt to move on from that history in the hope that a new generation might examine the ideas on their own merits. To do so, we must start with an overview of the common roots of both normalisation and SRV, the experiences, or 'wounds', of people who are devalued.

'Wounds' – description or label?

Students who adhere to the academic dictum of going to the original sources of ideas could do worse than try and discover a book called *Dehumanization and the Institutional Career* (Vail 1966). Wolfensberger, in his account of the early influences on normalisation noted above, gives prominence to this book as revealing, at least in public print and from the head of the Medical Services Division of a state Department of Public Welfare, the 'demeaning and debilitating' nature of institutions, then virtually the sole public provision. To our modern ears this seems so much common knowledge, as will the many references to Goffman's writings (1961, 1963) contained in Vail's book. As part of a pattern that was to be elaborated at much greater length and in many different forms, the reason I have highlighted this book is not so much its criticism of institutions (in fact its conclusions are really only aimed at making better institutions rather than doing away with them) but the notion of a 'career' of 'dehumanization', where both the environment and the way people are treated in that environment provide a series of what, to continue the analogy, we could call 'career milestones'. Unlike the more common usage of that term, to indicate steps onward, qualifications, more challenging jobs, etc., the career milestones of devalued people, particularly in the field of learning disability, tend to consist of negative experiences, reinforcing an identity that, as perceived by both the world and the person themselves, is also negative. From those seeds of normalisation, through to the formulation of SRV theory, the notion that individuals are 'wounded' by such experiences, and that attempts to address that wounding rely on reversing the process and the assumptions behind it, has, for me, been at the heart of all the variations, developments and reformulations. Regardless of the fact that devaluation was much more obvious in the large institutions, and was more clearly carried out in the case of people with learning difficulties, that core of wounding experiences identified back in the 1950s and 1960s still provides a powerful analysis of the lives of many devalued groups today, and is certainly one of the key reasons why I believe SRV is still relevant.

Space does not permit the detailed exposition of the depth of devaluation and wounding, which takes up a significant proportion of both Wolfensberger's (1998) and my own (1999a) accounts of SRV. Instead, the list of 'wounds' that I adapted for the latter work will be given in Table 11.1 below, and the question raised by critics and given at the heading of this section will be addressed, namely whether this description is, in itself, part of the devaluation process.

This analysis, which usually takes at least a full day when presented in SRV workshops, is a most powerful exposition of the relentlessness of devaluation. Other ways of describing these experiences were, as noted above, devised and used in PASS and PASSING workshops in the UK and elsewhere, most notably in the

Table 11.1 The most common experiences, or 'wounds', of devalued people

1   Impairment – physical and/or functional

    Leading to . . .

2   Relegation to low social status
3   Rejection, perhaps by family, neighbours, community, society
4   Cast into one or more devalued roles

4.1 As non-human	*4.2 As menaces, or objects of dread*
4.3 As waste, rubbish	*4.4 As trivium, or objects of ridicule*
4.5 As objects of pity	*4.6 As objects, or burden of charity*
4.7 As children	*4.8 As holy innocents*
4.9 As sick, or diseased	*4.10 In various death related roles*

    Which in turn usually results in . . .

5   Symbolic stigmatising – reinforcing the devalued perception
6   Jeopardy of being suspected of multiple deviances
7   Distantiation, usually via segregation and congregation

    Which commonly is accompanied by . . .

8   Loss of control, perhaps even of autonomy and freedom
9   Discontinuity with the physical environment and objects
10 Social and relationship discontinuity and even abandonment
11 Loss of natural, freely given relationships and substitution of artificial, 'paid for' ones
12 Deindividualisation
13 Involuntary material poverty
14 Impoverishment of experience, especially that of the typical, valued world
15 Exclusion from knowledge of and participation in higher-order value systems
16 Having one's life 'wasted'
17 Brutalisation – 'deathmaking'

    Which can give rise to the following feelings . . .

18 Awareness of being a source of anguish to those who love one
19 Awareness of being an alien in the valued world
20 Resentment, even hatred of privileged citizens

Source: Reproduced from Race (1999a: 44) – table adapted from Wolfensberger (1992).

telling of individual stories of people, and some of the accounts of life given by people with learning difficulties given elsewhere in this book are witness to the equally potent nature of this approach. In SRV workshops, however, where the full analysis is presented, the power comes from the detail and overwhelming nature of the wounds, their continuity and interconnectedness, and the ability of listeners to relate them to many real examples of vulnerable people. As presentations have developed over the years, the subtlety, too, of these elements of devaluation has been revealed. So, for example, the wound of distantiation, most obviously manifest in its roots in the analysis of institutionalisation, has many more recent and nuanced examples of people being put at a distance, even though they are 'in the community'. Similarly the wound of brutalisation and 'deathmaking', with its origins in the physical assaults and occasional fatalities in institutions, has its modern equivalents in the debate over genetic screening of 'defective' unborn children and the selective nature of hospital treatment to people with learning difficulties, (see e.g. Ryan and Thomas 1987, and the discussion in the last chapter of this book).

The other key factor in the wounds analysis is classification of the historic roles into which devalued people are cast. This, of course, had been around in normalisation, and forms one of the key parts of Wolfensberger's 1972 text, but it also led to the greater emphasis on roles as being key instruments in devaluation, which, in turn, informed the development of SRV. This will be discussed further below, but the issue must first be addressed of whether, by describing the wounds in this graphic and detailed way, SRV (and normalisation) are 'labelling' people as 'devalued' and thereby contributing to their oppression.

The issue has been at the heart of criticism of normalisation, especially by those who would see it (and SRV) as incompatible with ideas of self-determination and rights of disabled people, and at the academic level as being a theory at odds with the social theory of disability (see Chapter 12). I would contend that any response to this argument will really depend on a values position, not on rational analysis of empirical information. If one holds the view that *only* people's own definition of their situation is a valid one, then *any* external attempt to describe that situation will be declared invalid, still more so if that external attempt results in the sort of generalisation that Wolfensberger would describe as the 'universality' of wounding. If that rejection of external analysis is taken further to view all attempts to define need, or plan services or other responses to need, as being an 'imposition of other's views', then the wounds description would indeed be seen as oppressive, parallel to the 'personal tragedy' representation of disabled people so excoriated by the disability movement (e.g. Oliver 1990). It is, however, a values position, as it stems from the belief noted above.

A different position might be to see accounts of the lives of vulnerable people as having validity at an empirical level, i.e. to acknowledge that devaluation does occur, to judge the validity of the wounds analysis as a detailed description of the process that can be verified from experience and observation, and then to react to that according to one's values. Certainly the 'Problems facing learning disability services' in the *Valuing People* White Paper, especially under the sub-heading 'Social exclusion' have as many parallels in the wounds analysis as they do in the social theory of disability. Reaction to the 'problems' comes in ways which are also entirely compatible with strategies suggested by SRV, though the balance emphasises 'Rights, independence, choice and inclusion' with the obviously greater connection to O'Brien's 'Accomplishments' and the aims of the disability rights movement. The reality would seem to be that if any organised services are to exist for people with learning difficulties, then they will be based on a set of values largely articulated by others, however much people with learning difficulties have participated in the process, and that those values determine one's reaction to devaluation. To argue, therefore, that SRV's analysis of wounds contributes to devaluation would also be to argue that the White Paper's description of 'problems' contributes to devaluation, and thus that no attempt should be made by learning disability services to develop and change.

If, instead, one takes the view that devaluation exists, and that the description of wounds by SRV is as valid as any other empirical analysis of the phenomenon, then it is possible to go on to consider the weight that SRV gives to the concept of roles, and their place in valuation or devaluation.

Roles – the key to addressing devaluation or an interesting sideshow?

In his response to the opening addresses of Wolfensberger and Nirje at the 1994 Ottawa conference Michael Oliver, one of the foremost academics associated with the social theory of disability, admitted to not having read too much about normalisation, still less SRV (Oliver 1999). As well as going on to outline the social theory, Oliver's relative ignorance of SRV did not prevent him making a remark, common in the reaction of certain groups to ideas of 'deviancy theory' and 'role theory' that 'Not only are Talcott Parsons and Erving Goffman dead in a material sense but so are their products, the macro and micro versions of role theory' (Oliver, in Flynn and Lemay 1999: 171).

What he was accusing normalisation and SRV (and Wolfensberger personally) of not doing was producing a 'political' analysis of the situation of devalued people, something which certain sociologists in the UK, especially in the former polytechnics that Margaret Thatcher turned into universities, regarded not only as *a* way, but the only *true* way of analysing oppression. In this view those 'dead white male' sociologists who described the situation of devalued people in terms of their being cast into 'deviant roles' by society were outdated and 'functionalist', i.e. they implicitly supported the status quo by implying that devaluation came, as it were, 'naturally' by one section of society over another. This is contrasted with the 'historical materialism' of the Marxist approach common to Oliver and his fellow sociologists, who argue that only by the political and economic trans-formation of society will devaluation of disabled people, and all other 'different' groups be eradicated.

There are two key points for this chapter in their debate. One repeats the point made above, that they are, as with wounds, arguing from different values and belief positions, since the debate is essentially about what constitutes a better society. The second point is more academic, in the sense that Oliver's view of the demise of role theory along with some of its originators is not shared universally in academia (Radtke and Stam 1994). On the first point, the very title of this book, and certainly the overall philosophy outlined in the Introduction, is that learning disability is a socially generated phenomenon. Where this author would differ from Oliver, at least as far as SRV is concerned, is that I believe that people with learning difficulties can't wait for the revolution to have their oppression addressed and that as many means as possible should be brought to bear on society to do just that (including many of the suggestions proposed by Kathy Boxall in Chapter 12). Therefore SRV, though it comes from academia rather than disabled people, can be one of those strategies.

On the second point, rather than go into the process of counting academic references in favour of one position or the other, this chapter, as it did with the wounds, will simply present an overview of why roles seem to be important in devaluation and revaluation. Their relative importance in addressing devaluation, as distinct from, say, attempts to get legal rights for people with learning difficulties, will depend on readers' beliefs in the relative power of different strategies to achieve the 'good things of life' for people, of which more later.

So, to put it perhaps too simply, SRV posits that all people have roles in their society. Some of these are ascribed, i.e. they are given to a person by others, or by virtue of historical attribution. So the role of pupil in a school is ascribed by societies having created the whole institution of education, and demanding that children up to a certain age attend school, and act in the role of pupil. The role of son or daughter is ascribed by the simple and inescapable fact of being born. Other roles can be assumed by individuals, such as group leader, or employee, though in most cases assent by at least significant others to the role assumption is needed for the role to be a reality. Roles are ways in which members of any grouping of people, from a partnership up to a whole society, are afforded status and identity in that grouping. Along with that status and identity come expectations, the successful performance of which reinforces the role. This, of course, is where the nuancing of role expectations between different groups and sub-groups in society comes in, so that what is expected of one role by one group may differ from expectations of the same role by another group.

This is where, also, the power of different groups in society, both to define roles, and to define the expectations of them, impacts significantly on whether those roles are valued or devalued, and to what degree. So, in the wounds, reference back to Table 11.1 will remind us of the historical roles of devalued people, and a moment's thought should persuade us of how deeply imbedded in our societies many of those are (*pace* Oliver, they also seem to be embedded in both capitalist and socialist societies, as well as in pre-industrialised societies). It also, to me, is where SRV and the social theory of disability come closest together, in that those roles are socially imposed, and result in the oppression of disabled people, as they do of many other vulnerable groups. Where the difference comes, as between SRV and other strategies such as inclusion, is what one then does about the phenomenon. SRV proposes that the power of role expectancy is then used to counter devaluation, by trying to get people out of devalued roles (especially the historically embedded ones) and into valued roles. This, however, is described by Wolfensberger (1998) as a 'second order' goal of SRV. The 'primary' goal needs to be discussed first, namely the 'good things of life' for devalued and vulnerable people.

The goals of SRV

Throughout this chapter the intrusion of values issues at every stage has been inevitable. Inevitable because we are not just talking about competing technologies to reach agreed ends, but the lives of real people. In examining Table 11.2, therefore (adapted from work by Wolfensberger and others), readers are invited not only to compare how many of the indicators they themselves aspire to, but to return to the lives of people with learning difficulties dispersed throughout this book, and note how similar are their aspirations for such things, and how common is their deprivation of many of them.The language of Table 11.2 again has echoes in the 'Principles' of the 2001 White Paper, and, I would argue, places the primary goal of SRV as complementary to the goals of that document. Going on to the secondary goal, that used in the 1995 definition of SRV, namely the 'enablement, establishment, maintenance and/or defence of valued roles for people', we can again find many parallels. Out of the eleven objectives given in the White Paper (p. 26) the seven that are expressed in terms of outcomes for people with learning difficulties (as opposed to others for carers and the services) all can be expressed in terms of roles. Opportunities for children, for example, to fill the valued role of pupil in regular education (from Objective 1). Or for adults to fill the valued role of home owner or tenant (from Objective 6) or worker in open employment (from

Table 11.2 The 'good things in life' – the primary goal of SRV for devalued people

Family, or small intimate group	A place to call home
An intermediate but still small-scale social group	Friends
A transcendent belief system	Work, especially meaningful work
Absence of imminent threats of extreme privation	Opportunities and expectations to discover and develop skills, abilities, gifts and talents
To be viewed as a human and treated with respect	To be dealt with honestly
To be treated justly	To be treated as an individual
To have a say in important issues affecting one's life	Access to most of the 'sites of everyday life'
Access to at least many of the activities of human social life	Being able to contribute, and having one's contributions recognised as valuable
Good health	

Source: reproduced from Race (1999a: 97) – table adapted from Wolfensberger *et al.* (1996).

Objective 8). Still more relevant are the many roles covered by the part of Objective 7 that aims to 'develop a range of friendships, activities and relationships'.

Once we get to this point in the goals of SRV, the theory suggests strategies within its own framework to achieve them. This is the point at which SRV's strategies can be compared with other means to achieve at least the primary goal of achieving the good things of life for people. SRV theory uses the framework of PASSING (see Chapter 7) to divide its strategies and sub-strategies into two main groupings, namely those affecting a group or individual's *social image*, and those affecting their *competency*. Those two sub-headings then provide a focus for action along one or a number of what have been called the 'channels' through which role messages and role expectancies are conveyed. These are summarised in Table 11.3.

Table 11.3 Major channels through which role messages and role expectancies are conveyed

1	Physical environments	(a)	Structure, i.e the physical design and features
		(b)	Context, i.e the location, proximity to other settings, history and access of a setting
2	Social context	(a)	The people or groups associated with the group or person – in a service context, the people sharing the same service
		(b)	The people or groups physically near the group or person – in a service context this may be service staff, or users of other services located nearby
3	Activities		Behaviours carried out by, expected or demanded of a person or group, including the nature and timing of those activities
4	Language	(a)	Language directly addressed to a person or group
		(b)	Language used indirectly about a person or group
		(c)	Names of services and service settings
		(d)	Language and other symbols connected to a person or group by referring to their activities, service processes or other people or groups that they are associated with or near to
5	Personal presentation	(a)	The posture, bodily appearance and expressive movement
		(b)	Clothes and other personal attire
		(c)	Grooming
		(d)	Other distinguishing marks, e.g. tattoos, insignia
		(e)	Possessions
6	Miscellaneous aspects		e.g. Source of funding of services

Source: reproduced from Race (1999a: 93) – table adapted from Wolfensberger and Thomas (1983).

In an overview of this kind, it is difficult to convey the rich tapestry of possibilities that such strategies offer. What is important to stress here is the variety of *levels* of social organisation at which they can be applied, addressing the commonly expressed criticism that SRV is all about 'moulding individuals' to 'fit' into society. While there certainly are efforts that can be made at the individual level, to enhance both an individual's image and competency, Wolfensberger has always taught, even in the application of normalisation, that action is also possible, and may well have a more beneficial effect for groups of people, at the level of primary or intermediate social systems and even of entire societies (see Wolfensberger 1972, table I: 32 for an early published example of this point). Arranging, or working to arrange, the physical and social conditions of a small group for example, so that their image is that of a group of valued citizens, participating in their local communities with valued roles such as householder or worker, can do much to increase the probability that the whole group, not just certain individuals, will be afforded some of the good things of life. Arranging the social and physical conditions of services for, say, elderly people in a locality so that the image of those people does not cast them into the death or dying roles, can have major effects on the whole elderly population. Working towards policies and legislation, such as those of the White Paper, which would increase the access to employment of people with learning difficulties and thereby enhance their image as contributing citizens could have effects on the value afforded to people with learning difficulties as a whole. All of the above are examples of action possibilities suggested by SRV at different societal levels to enhance people's image, which is crucial to how people are perceived, and therefore to what roles they hold or are given, and therefore their vulnerability to devaluation. Action at all levels is equally important within SRV theory, at least in the sense that SRV would not suggest stopping work with individuals because society hasn't changed, or not working with a group because all the individuals in it might not benefit equally.

The same applies to efforts to enhance people's competency. Arranging the physical and social conditions so that an individual's competencies are likely to be enhanced is a powerful tool in increasing the valued roles played by that individual, but there are efforts that can equally be made within the primary and intermediate social systems to which people belong, and even at the whole society level. Whatever one thinks of the 'lifelong learning' initiative of the current government, for example, it has afforded many people and groups the opportunity to increase their competencies in certain areas, and therefore take up, or be perceived in, more valued roles. So, with the clear understanding that they can take place at all levels of society, such efforts can therefore take their place in the broader range of strategies for establishing valued roles for people, the secondary goal of SRV. As a generality, one would want both to mould the roles that people or groups might play so that they are seen as positive by observers and to affect the values held by others so as to value, or at least not devalue, characteristics and roles that people or groups already hold. The means to do this are more likely to succeed if they themselves are culturally valued. This means being aware, again at all levels, of what is seen as age-appropriate and culture appropriate and appreciating the subtle nuances and changes in those social judgements.

Within SRV theory teaching, and also in the longer published works mentioned above, the foregoing analysis of the goals of SRV is followed by a further aid to understanding the complexity and subtlety of the theory in practice, namely what are referred to as the 'themes' of SRV. Again, readers are referred to those publications for such detail. For the purposes of this chapter the overview of SRV will close here, with a conclusion on the chapter's main issues.

Conclusion – moving on

The main effort of this chapter has been twofold. One, to try and give the reader some inkling as to the way in which a set of ideas, called 'normalisation', came, had a major impact, and yet whose development into SRV was, and is, poorly addressed in this country, both in academia and in the world of services. Two, by relating SRV theory, at least in outline and in terms of its major goals, to learning disability services, and especially the White Paper, the attempt is made to convince the reader, whether they are from either or none of the groups above, that further study of SRV has something to offer in addressing the devaluation which both it and its predecessor identify so clearly, and which other parts of this book illustrate in a variety of different ways. It was, and is, clearly possible, given the number of contributors to this book who worked alongside my own teaching of SRV on the degree course at Stockport, for a range of views to be presented within a degree course that others seem to think totally incompatible. One therefore hopes that the UK academic and service world will not be so tied up by their history that they cannot see a place for SRV within efforts to improve learning disability services, and will therefore 'move on' from endless replays of the normalisation debate.

References

Alaszewski, A. and Ong, B.N. (eds) (1990) *Normalisation in Practice: Residential Care for Children with a Profound Mental Handicap*, London, Routledge.

Brown, H. and Smith, H. (1992) *Normalisation – a Reader for the Nineties*, London, Routledge.

Emerson, E. (1992) What is normalization? In: H. Brown and H. Smith (eds), *Normalization – a Reader for the Nineties*, London, Routledge.

Flynn, R.J. and Lemay, R.A. (eds) (1999) *A Quarter Century of Normalization and Social Role Valorization: Evolution and Impact*, Ottawa, University of Ottawa Press.

Gates, R. (1997), *Learning Disabilities, 3rd edition*, New York, Edinburgh, Churchill Livingstone.

Goffman, E. (1961) *Asylums – Essays on the Social Situation of Mental Patients and Other Inmates*, Gordon City, NY, Doubleday.

Goffman, E. (1963) *Stigma: Notes on the Management of Spoiled Identity*, New York, Prentice-Hall.

Harper, G. (1990) A better life on the outside, *Community Living*, 3(4): 14–16.

Lyle O'Brien, C. and O'Brien, J. (2000) *The Origins of Person-centred Planning: A Community of Practice Perspective*, Georgia, Responsive Systems Associates.

Millier, P. (1999) Normalization and social role valorization in Australia and New Zealand. In: R.J. Flynn and R.A. Lemay (eds) *A Quarter Century of Normalization and Social Role Valorization: Evolution and Impact*, Ottawa, University of Ottawa Press.

O'Brien, J. (1985) *Normalization training through PASS3: Team Leader Manual*, Decatur GA, USA, Responsive Systems Associates.

O'Brien, J. (1987) A guide to personal futures planning. In: G. Bellamy and B. Wilcox (eds), *A Comprehensive Guide to the Activities Catalogue: An Alternative Curriculum for Youth and Adults with Severe Disabilities*, Baltimore, Paul Brookes.

O'Brien J (1999) Education in applying the principle of normalization as a factor in the practical arts of improving services for socially devalued people. In: R.J. Flynn and R.A. Lemay (eds) *A Quarter Century of Normalization and Social Role Valorization: Evolution and Impact*, Ottawa, University of Ottawa Press.

O'Brien, J. and O'Brien, C. (1989) *Framework for Accomplishment Workshop Manual*, Georgia, Responsive Systems Associates.

Oliver, M. (1990) *The Politics of Disablement*, London, Macmillan.

Oliver M.J. (1999) Capitalism, disability and ideology: a materialist critique of the Normalization principle. In: R.J. Flynn and R.A. Lemay (eds) *A Quarter Century of Normalization and Social Role Valorization: Evolution and Impact*, Ottawa, University of Ottawa Press.

Race, D.G. (1999a) *Social Role Valorization and the English Experience*, Wilding and Birch, London.

Race, D.G. (1999b) Hearts and minds: Social Role Valorization, UK academia and services for people with a learning disability, *Disability and Society*, 14(4): 519–538.

Radtke, H.L. and Stam, H. (eds) (1994) *Power/Gender: Social Relations in Theory and Practice*, London, Sage.

Ramcharan, P., Roberts, G., Grant, G. and Borland, J. (eds) (1997) *Empowerment in Everyday life: Learning Disability*, London, Jessica Kingsley.

Ryan, J. and Thomas, F. (1987) *The Politics of Mental Handicap (2nd edition)*, Harmondsworth, Penguin.

Tyne, A. (1994) Taking responsibility and Giving Power, *Disability and Society*, 9(2): 249–54.

Vail, D.J. (1966) *Dehumanization and the Institutional Career*, Springfield, IL, Charles C. Thomas.

Wolfensberger, W. (1972) *The Principle of Normalization in Human Services*, Toronto, NIMR.

Wolfensberger, W. (1983) Social Role Valorization: A proposed new term for the principle of normalization, *Mental Retardation*, 21: 234–239.

Wolfensberger, W. (1984) A reconceptualization of Normalization as Social Role Valorization, *Canadian Journal on Mental Retardation*, 34(2): 22–26.

Wolfensberger, W. (1985) Social Role Valorization: A new insight, and a new term, for Normalization, *Australian Association for the Mentally Retarded Journal*, 9(1): 4–11.

Wolfensberger, W. (1989a) Human service policy: The rhetoric versus the reality. In: L. Barton (ed.), *Disability and Dependency*, London, Falmer Press.

Wolfensberger, W. (1989b) *The New Genocide of Handicapped and Afflicted People*, Syracuse, NY, Training Institute for Human Services Planning, Leadership and Change Agentry, Syracuse University.

Wolfensberger, W. (1992) *A Brief Introduction to Social Role Valorization as a High Order Concept for Structuring Human Services, 2nd edition* (revised), Syracuse NY, Training Institute for Human Service Planning, Leadership and Change Agentry, Syracuse University.

Wolfensberger, W. (1998) *A Brief Introduction to Social Role Valorization: a High Order Concept for Addressing the Plight of Societally Devalued People, and for Structuring Human Services, 3rd edition* (revised), Syracuse NY, Training Institute for Human Services Planning, Leadership and Change Agentry, Syracuse University.

Wolfensberger, W. (1999a) A contribution to the history of Normalization, with primary emphasis on the establishment of Normalization in North America between 1967–1975. In: R.J. Flynn and R.A. Lemay (eds) *A Quarter Century of Normalization and Social Role Valorization: Evolution and Impact*, Ottawa, University of Ottawa Press.

Wolfensberger, W. (1999b) Concluding reflections and a look ahead into the future for Normalization and Social Role Valorization. In: R.J. Flynn and R.A. Lemay (eds) *A Quarter Century of Normalization and Social Role Valorization: Evolution and Impact*. Ottawa, University of Ottawa Press.

Wolfensberger, W. and Glenn, L. (1975) *Program Analysis of Service Systems (PASS): a method for the quantitative evaluation of human services 3rd edition, Vol. I: Handbook. Vol II: Field Manual*, Toronto, NIMR.

Wolfensberger, W. and Thomas, S. (1983) *Program Analysis of Service Systems' Implementations of Normalization Goals (PASSING)*, Toronto, NIMR.

Wolfensberger, W., Thomas, S. and Caruso, G. (1996), Some of the universal 'good things in life' which the implementation of Social Role Valorization can be expected to make more accessible to devalued people, *International Social Role Valorization Journal*, 2(2): 12–14.

Chapter 12

Individual and social models of disability and the experiences of people with learning difficulties

Kathy Boxall

Introduction

This chapter examines some of the discussions about disability which have been taking place within the disabled people's movement and considers the relevance of these ideas to people identified as having learning difficulties. Within the UK disabled people's movement, ideas of disability are frequently framed in terms of *individual* and *social* models of disability. These two diametrically opposed models appear to offer an illuminating universal tool to aid understanding and analysis of disability. Some disabled people have, however, criticised the formulaic simplicity of such an approach and point to its lack of sophistication in accounting for their individual experiences (see, for example, Morris 1991, 1996; Crow 1996; Vernon 1998). Other disabled people have challenged such critiques for fragmenting the coherence offered to the disabled people's movement by a unifying social model of disability (for example, Oliver 1996a; Barnes 1998).

A number of authors have made links between these critical discourses and the relevance of the social model of disability to people with learning difficulties (Chappell 1998; Goodley 2000, 2001; Dowse 2001). Before going on to examine some of these critiques, I wish first to present straightforward summaries of the medical, individual and social models of disability and relate these to the experiences of people identified as having learning difficulties.

The medical model of disability

Though reference is sometimes made to a *medical model* of disability, there is little in the literature which specifically defines a medical model approach. Deborah Marks (1999: 52) suggests that this is because the term 'tends only to be employed by those critical of medical practices. Doctors tend not to see themselves as "proponents of the medical model".' She goes on to offer a definition of the medical model which centres around the concept of *disease*: a temporary organic state which is experienced by a sick individual who then becomes the object of medical treatment aimed at eradicating that disease. This approach is based upon the scientific understanding of the human body as a biological or physiological system.

In medical model terms, disability is an individual functional limitation (something the individual 'can't do', or has 'wrong' with them) *which has a biological or physiological cause*. Biomedical diagnosis locates the 'problem' of disability in the individual, and emphasises his/her individual pathology and personal deficit. In this way, disability is viewed as 'personal tragedy' (Oliver 1990). The medical model response to diagnosis of illness, disease or disability is *individual medical treatment*. Some disabled people have, however, objected to the inappropriateness of this medicalisation of their experience because 'their impairments, even if they were disease-based, were not amenable to being *cured* by medical advances' (Oliver and Barnes 1998: 7, emphasis added).

Simon Brisenden, a disabled activist and writer, argued that because of its claim to expertise in the diagnosis and treatment of disability, the medical profession's response to disabled people is, of necessity, bounded:

> doctors and others are trapped in their responses by a definition of their own making. They cannot respond in ways that go outside the parameters of a view of disabled people which they themselves have created. They are stuck within a medical model of disability.
>
> (Brisenden 1998 [1986]: 24)

This medical model view of disabled people also serves to position disability firmly within the domain of the medical profession and the bounds of its professional power (Wilding 1982).

The medical model and people with learning difficulties

The influence of medical model approaches is evident in the historical treatment of people with learning difficulties, as detailed in Chapter 2. As late as the 1950s, people were diagnosed as 'idiots', 'imbeciles', 'mental or moral defectives' and incarcerated in long-stay institutions or 'colonies' under the eugenically motivated Mental Deficiency Act 1913 (Potts and Fido 1991; Thomson 1998). Two medical practitioners were required to certify an individual 'a fit person to be removed' to an institution. They did this by asking the individual a series of general knowledge questions and listing 'wrong answers' as evidence of 'mental deficiency':

> He fails to form a sentence with three given words. He fails to multiply by seven, to state the number of half-crowns in 15s. And to correct a slow clock. He fails to state similarities in an apple and an orange, to repeat five digits backwards and to solve a simple test of reasoning.
>
> (Potts and Fido 1991: 19)

David Barron (2001) cites a similar example from his own medical records.

He cannot read or write, or state the months of the year. Cannot add 24 and 6. Does not know how many pence there are in 8/6. He has no general knowledge. (1932, age 7 years).

Maggie Potts and Rebecca Fido (1991) point to the marked contrast between the questions asked in the certification process and the type of education (if any) received by 'defective' children. This is borne out by David Barron's (2001) description of his lack of tuition in the 'three Rs' in the special school he attended prior to being institutionalised.

Despite the apparent lack of objective scientific measures, perceived 'defect' was deemed 'pathological' and condemned the individual to a negative and overly pessimistic 'prognosis'.

Low-grade defect appears to be almost invariably determined by pathological abnormalities, related, in various ways, to such low mental (and often other) potentials, that the most humane and devoted care, supplemented by all available scientific resources, cannot bring the social prognosis of idiots and most imbeciles within the socially tolerable range.

(MacMahon 1955, cited by O'Connor and Tizard 1956: 155)

In medical model terms, the 'problem' was mental deficiency or, more particularly, the *individual pathology* of 'defectives'. The medical model 'solution' was the *colony*. Individual defectives were removed from society and placed in colonies where segregation of the sexes was strictly enforced so that they could be prevented from 'repeating their type' (Potts and Fido 1991 and see again Chapter 2 of this book).

Mathew Thomson regards the Mental Deficiency Act 1913 as an example of professional imperialism on the part of the medical profession and argues that it may be interpreted as:

providing a further outlet for professional expansion, creating a new class of deviants in need of control, and adopting hereditarian arguments to highlight the urgency of the problem and the need for medical management.

(Thomson 1998: 111)

The individual model of disability

Michael Oliver (1996b: 31) maintains that 'there is no such thing as the medical model of disability, there is instead, an individual model of disability of which medicalisation is one significant component'. From an *individual model* perspective, disability is a tragic problem for isolated individuals. Once diagnosed or identified as disabled, individuals are offered ameliorative 'treatment' or 'rehabilitation' which may (or may not) be medically based.

The individual model presumes that 'disability' takes over the individual's identity and constrains 'unrealistic' hopes and ambitions . . . individuals are socialised into a traditional disabled role and identity, and expected to submit to professional intervention in order to facilitate their adjustment to their 'personal tragedy'.

(Barnes *et al.* 1999: 26)

Professional intervention may be from a range of medical or *non-medical* professionals including social workers, educational psychologists, teachers and employment rehabilitation workers. On a wider scale, individual model responses may result in policies that continue to locate the 'problem' of disability in the individual and fail to consider external causes.

Colin Barnes points to the Chronically Sick and Disabled Persons Act 1970 and the establishment of Local Authority Social Services Departments in the early 1970s as a watershed in terms of the numbers of different professionals involved in disabled people's lives. 'This resulted in a situation where almost every aspect of life for a disabled person had its counterpart in a profession or voluntary organisation' (Barnes 1991: 23).

The individual model and people with learning difficulties

Individual model approaches are apparent within the special education system for children with learning difficulties. Prior to 1971, many children with more 'severe' or 'profound' learning difficulties were, following assessment, deemed 'ineducable' and had no entitlement to an education. In individual model terms, the 'problem' was the 'ineducable' child. For some parents, with the exception of placing their child in a long-stay hospital, no 'solution' was offered. Others were offered discretionary places in 'Hospital Schools' or 'Junior Training Centres'. Doreen Lakin (2000) describes the excitement she felt when in 1967, following assessment by a Mental Health Officer, she was told that her daughter Melanie could have such a place.

In 1971, the Education (Handicapped Children) Act 1970 came into force and children with 'severe' or 'profound' learning difficulties were for the first time afforded the right to an education. Following assessment, children like Melanie were placed in schools specifically for 'Educationally Subnormal (Severe)' or 'ESN(S)' children (Tomlinson 1982). Although viewed positively at the time, this individual model approach located the 'problem' within the child. The individual model 'solution' or 'treatment' for that child was *segregated special education* (see the discussion in Chapter 4).

The social model of disability

Unlike the individual model of disability which locates the 'problem' of disability in the individual, the social model of disability views disability as 'a situation of collective institutional discrimination and social oppression' (Oliver and Barnes 1998: 3). The social model of disability is concerned with the *barriers* within our society which serve to *disable* people with impairments. From a social model perspective, disability is not caused by people's impairments: it is the failures of society to accommodate people with impairments that cause disability. In other words, disability is viewed 'as a social state, rather than as a biological difference' (Barnes *et al.* 1999: 37).

According to the social model, people who use wheelchairs are *disabled* by contemporary social organisation that takes little or no account of wheelchair users. On the front cover of Michael Oliver's (1990) *The Politics of Disablement* there is a photograph of a wheelchair user at the bottom of a flight of steps leading to a Polling Station. This disabled man experiences disadvantage and discrimination because of the *physical barriers* (steps) which are there to facilitate the access of non-disabled voters but which prevent him from entering the building. He may also experience *attitudinal barriers*. Because he is a wheelchair user, non-disabled officials, professionals, members of the public, relatives or friends may assume he is unable to be independent and may place restrictions on the everyday control he exercises over his own life. Such restrictions extend to policies that control the type of education he received as a child and the way in which he can exercise his right to vote as an adult. He is also likely to be disadvantaged within the labour market and to experience poverty (Oliver 1990, 1996b; Barnes 1991; Oliver and Barnes 1998). In social model terms, it is these *barriers* which cause him to experience disablement. If it were possible to remove all physical and attitudinal barriers, wheelchair users would no longer be disabled in our society. Conversely, it is possible for other (previously non-disabled) people to experience disablement if the environment and wider social structures are organised in such a way as to create barriers to their full and active participation in society.

This is illustrated by Vic Finkelstein's (1981) imaginary wheelchair village that was organised for the benefit and convenience of the wheelchair users who lived there. Finkelstein's wheelchair user villagers designed village buildings to suit their physical needs with ramps and lower doors and ceilings than would normally be found in the non-disabled world. They also organised employment within the village in such a way that it met the needs of wheelchair users. As a result, the wheelchair user villagers did not experience disablement within their village. However, a small number of 'able-bodied' people settled in the village and, as a result of the lowered doors and ceilings, experienced difficulties in using the buildings. They became known as 'the able-bodied disabled' and were treated in a similar way to disabled people in our disablist society. They received 'treatment' for their bruised heads and were fitted with helmets and special braces which bent them double in order to prevent them injuring themselves. They also experienced discrimination in the labour market and charitable organisations were set up by the wheelchair user villagers in order to provide for the needs of the 'able-bodied disabled'.

The social model and people with learning difficulties

When considering the social model in relation to people with learning difficulties, there are a number of parallels with the examples relating to physical impairment above. People with learning difficulties may experience similar attitudinal barriers and subsequent loss of independence and control over their own lives. There are also issues of access, particularly access to information presented in formats which may be inaccessible to many people with learning difficulties, for example written or verbal language containing jargon or big words (Aspis 1999). People with learning difficulties also experience discrimination within the education system (Murray and Penman 1996, 2000 and see Chapter 4) and the labour market (Baron *et al.* 1998; DoH 2001 and see Chapter 5). According to the social model of disability, if these barriers could be removed by changing attitudes and making information more accessible, people with learning difficulties would be less disabled in our society.

Within the education system, some children with learning difficulties, particularly those who have 'profound' learning difficulties or those identified as having challenging behaviours, continue to be educated in segregated 'special schools' ostensibly because it isn't possible to meet the child's needs within a mainstream school setting. This individual model assessment locates the 'problem' within the individual child. Assessment from a social model perspective, however, would locate the 'problem' within the education system rather than the child. Instead of considering the child with learning difficulties to have 'failed', it would consider the 'failure' of the mainstream school environment to accommodate the needs of that child. It would also consider the education policies, local and national, which fail to promote mainstream provision for *some* children with learning difficulties. A social model approach to educating a child with learning difficulties would entail looking at the mainstream school environment and considering ways of modifying that environment so that the child's educational needs could be met within that setting.

The following examples, taken from a collection of stories compiled by Pippa Murray and Jill Penman illustrate differences between individual model and social model approaches:

> for two years we've been trying to explain that it is the school that must change and not the child. It seems the school cannot understand.
>
> It is explained to us that children must be able to sit still, be quiet, concentrate, not disrupt other children: to 'progress' in order to move on with their peers.
>
> 'He can't sit still', I explain. 'I've said this all along. You can't expect him to. He needs support with this. That is how he is.'
>
> . . . It makes me want to keep him completely out of the system as it is today.
>
> ('Name withheld', in Murray and Penman 1996: 73)

A more positive example is provided by Julie Dalton's description of her daughter Jen's first term at mainstream school. She describes how Jen was supported by her 'special friend' Sam in the school Nativity Play:

> Her teacher had asked me to help Jen memorise three lines that she was going to say with two other children, one being Sam. I could not imagine in a month of Sundays Jen being able to do this in front of other people, or knowing when to stand up or sit down, but there she was on the front row. Sam gave her a prod when to stand up and also told her when to sit down. The children also told her to 'shhh' when she started to get fidgety.
>
> (Julie Dalton in Murray and Penman 1996: 35)

The first example illustrates an individual model approach where the school has located the 'problem' within the child and wants the child to change; or be educated elsewhere. The second example, which could be described as a social model approach, illustrates how Jen's mainstream school has supported her by modifying the mainstream provision in order to accommodate Jen's educational needs. Within the mainstream classroom, Jen has a support worker. On this occasion, she was also given additional support by her teacher, mother and other children in her class. Her mother also explains that Jen is much loved by her friend Sam and is described by the school as being an 'asset' to the class (Julie Dalton in Murray and Penman 1996).

The example above of an imaginary wheelchair users' village (Finkelstein 1981) demonstrates how non-disabled people are *disabled* by the village environment. Kurt Vonnegut's (1969) science fiction story 'Harrison Bergeron' describes a society where people *without* learning difficulties are obliged to wear 'mental handicap radio' ear pieces. These are tuned to a government transmitter that periodically broadcasts loud noises in order to prevent wearers from concentrating for sustained periods. Though this story produces an interesting slant on equalising intellectual ability, the way in which it does this is not analogous to the wheelchair users' village example. Finkelstein's village is organised for the benefit and convenience of wheelchair users: their *advantage* is non-disabled people's *disadvantage*. An equivalent analogy would be a situation *which advantaged people with learning difficulties* whilst at the same time disadvantaging people without learning difficulties. It would be interesting to imagine such a scenario, though it would perhaps best be developed by people who themselves have lived experience of discrimination on the basis of identified 'learning difficulties'.

Social model terminology and people with learning difficulties

As David Race notes in the Introduction to this book, the UK disabled people's movement makes a clear distinction between *impairment* and *disability*. As Jenny Morris explains, this has important implications for the words used to identify or refer to people:

> Disability refers to the oppression which people with ... impairments experience as a result of prejudicial attitudes and discriminatory actions. People are disabled by society's reaction to impairment; this is why the term *disabled people* is used, rather than *people with disabilities* ... the disability movement prefers to use the politically more powerful term, *disabled people*, in order to place the emphasis on how society oppresses people with a whole range of impairments.
>
> (Morris 1993: x)

On this analysis, because people with learning difficulties also experience 'oppression as a result of prejudicial attitudes and discriminatory actions', they too are *disabled people*. Simone Aspis has written about her experiences of oppression and describes herself as 'a disabled person who has been labelled by the system as having learning difficulties' (1999: 174).

The term 'people with learning *disabilities*' is, however, more usually used in official circles and publications (for example DoH 2001). Referring to people in this way appears to indicate that 'disability' is located in the individual rather than in the wider social structures and environment. As Fran Branfield explains:

> Disablist ideologies claim that we are disabled by our impairments. A social model perspective, in contrast, holds that we are disabled by an uncaring and unjust society. This view leads inextricably to the fact that we cannot use terms or phrases such as 'people with disabilities' or 'learning disabilities' ... [as] such phrases become meaningless ... Quite simply then, a disability is not something an individual can own, it is something that is done to us by an oppressive society.
>
> (Branfield 2000: 371)

This issue of terminology is far from straightforward and is further complicated by the fact that disabled people's organisations outside the UK use the term *people with disabilities* (see for example Davis 1997) rather than *disabled people*. Terminology relating to 'intellectual impairment' also varies across continents.

However, within the UK authors writing from a social model perspective tend to use the term 'people with learning *difficulties*' in preference to the term 'people with learning *disabilities*'.

In the preface of his recent book on self-advocacy, Dan Goodley (2000) explains that this is because it is the term preferred by many in the self-advocacy movement. He cites a number of reports and publications by self-advocacy groups in Huddersfield, Liverpool and London which support this view and quotes one self-advocate who stated:

> 'If you put "people with learning difficulties" then they know that people want to learn and to be taught how to do things.'
>
> (Sutcliffe and Simons 1993: 23, cited by Goodley 2000: xiii)

The social model of disability and its critics

A number of disabled people have criticised the social model of disability, arguing that it does not adequately account for their experiences. For example, Liz Crow (1996) has argued that the social model's focus on the socially situated nature of disability relegates disabled people's experiences of impairment. For some disabled people, 'pain, fatigue, chronic illness and depression are constant facts of life' yet, in social model analysis, people's impairments are often regarded as irrelevant or neutral (Crow 1996: 209). Similarly, Sally French (1993) maintains that she is disabled partly *because of* her visual impairment, not simply because of 'socially imposed restriction'. Jenny Morris (1991, 1996) has argued that the social model has tended to marginalise disabled women's experiences and Ayesha Vernon (1998) has highlighted the marginalisation of other groups, for example Black disabled people, lesbians and gay men who are disabled, older disabled people and disabled people from the working class. Other authors (Chappell 1998; Goodley 2000, 2001; Dowse 2001) have made links between the situation of people with learning difficulties and these critical discussions, arguing that people with learning difficulties are similarly marginalised within the social model of disability. For example, Anne Louise Chappell suggests that:

> It appears the best that people with learning difficulties can expect is an implicit inclusion in any writing about disability. Thus some of the arguments emanating from within the social model are assumed to refer to *all* disabled people, when in reality they do not. Such arguments are clearly very partial.
>
> (Chappell 1998: 213–214)

Although the experiences of people with learning difficulties have often, as Chappell rightly points out, been excluded from social model discussion, it isn't necessarily the case that 'arguments emanating from the social model' do not apply to people with learning difficulties. It is possible that the partial nature of these arguments may have more to do with the lack of application of the social model to people with learning difficulties, than any failures on the part of the social model to account for their experiences.

The social model arose out of disabled people's lived experiences. It was developed as a reaction to non-disabled people's (mostly professionals and academics) ideas about disability and disabled people. A key aspect of social model theorising is that it has been both authored and controlled by disabled people themselves. As Fran Branfield has argued:

> the disability movement reflects a socio-political reality. For disabled people, this reality is immediate, growing out of our lived experience and producing direct knowledge for change, for action. 'Non-disabled' people cannot fully know this. For them, their experience, their history, their culture is our oppression.
>
> (Branfield 1998: 143–144)

With the notable exception of Simone Aspis (1999) there has been little contribution to social model literature by people with learning difficulties themselves. Where people with learning difficulties' experience *is* included in social model discussion, this is often in the form of their *researched* experience; researched and interpreted by people *without* learning difficulties. Where reference is made to people with learning difficulties' own published accounts of their experiences, these are then analysed by authors *without* learning difficulties. Consequently, literature relating the social model to the experiences of people with learning difficulties is largely being authored and controlled by people *without* learning difficulties. The majority of social model literature more generally, however, has been produced by disabled people (without learning difficulties) who, in the main, have not sought to represent the experiences of people identified as having learning difficulties. This is perhaps not surprising given the disabled people's movement's emphasis on *self*-representation and speaking on their own behalf.

Meanwhile, authors *without* learning difficulties are continuing to write about people with learning difficulties and the social model. It feels somewhat inappropriate that discussion about people with learning difficulties and an *emancipatory* social model of disability (Campbell and Oliver 1996) does not include the very people it claims to emancipate. There are also issues of ownership of that debate. If people without learning difficulties (myself included) author and control debate in this area, there is a risk that such discussion will form part of the process that problematises and constructs and reinforces the 'otherness' of the group being debated (Branfield 1998, 2000). A perhaps more apposite way of progressing such debate would be ask how people with learning difficulties could be better supported to represent *their own experiences* or develop *their own ideas* about the social model of disability and its relevance to their lives. If indeed that is what they want to do. Related to this, Chappell *et al.* (2001: 49) suggest that people with learning difficulties may already be '"doing" the social model although not writing about it or articulating it in a theoretical language'. They argue that it is crucial that researchers develop innovative ways of researching this 'doing' of the social model.

This is something that Dan Goodley explores in relation to self-advocacy. He draws upon a range of literature and resources produced by people with learning difficulties, including the 'life stories of top self-advocates' who participated in his research. Goodley also proposes an 'inclusive' social model of disability which makes links with academic literature relating to the social construction of 'learning difficulties'. He argues that 'the social model of disability can only include people with learning difficulties when it recognises the social origins of "learning difficulties" and "difference"' (Goodley 2000: 36). Goodley's inclusive social model appears to blur the distinction between 'impairment' and 'disability' in that he views both as socially constructed when related to people with learning difficulties.

This position differs markedly from that of disabled people such as Liz Crow (1996) who view the 'pain, fatigue, chronic illness and depression' of their impairments as far from socially constructed. Other disabled people, for example

Michael Oliver (1996a) and Colin Barnes (1998), have argued that criticism of the social model which focuses on the pain and distress of impairment has strong similarities with individual model approaches. Such criticism:

> may not broaden and refine the social model; it may instead breathe new life in the individual model with all that means in terms of increasing medical and therapeutic interventions into areas of our lives where they do not belong.
>
> (Oliver 1996a: 52)

Individual model approaches have not served people with learning difficulties very well (see for example Ryan and Thomas 1987; Potts and Fido 1991; and much of this book). It is important therefore that critical discussions of the social model of disability and people with learning difficulties avoid 'breathing new life into the individual model'. Rather than focusing on the marginalisation of people with learning difficulties within the social model of disability, it may be preferable to look at ways in which people with learning difficulties could be supported to contribute to social model discussions. I have outlined below a number of suggestions for supporting the development of such discussions:

Drawing upon people with learning difficulties' own literature, materials and resources

Some people with learning difficulties have documented their experiences and a number of these accounts have achieved publication (including, of course, in this book). Paul Williams (1999) identifies existing literature by people who have Down's syndrome and Dan Goodley (2000) points to other sources produced by people with learning difficulties. These include Nigel Hunt's (1967) autobiography and an edited collection of people with learning difficulties' work (Atkinson and Williams 1990). Other examples are David Barron's (1996) autobiography, which was originally published privately in the 1980s, and a recent edited collection of experiences of disability which includes contributions by people with learning difficulties (Murray and Penman 2000). It is possible that there are other documented sources by people with learning difficulties, as yet unpublished.

Supporting people with learning difficulties to record their own experiences or life stories

There are several examples of oral history projects which record the personal histories of people with learning difficulties, for example Potts and Fido (1991) and Atkinson et al. (1997). These provide a rich source of the *lived experiences* of people identified as having learning difficulties. Some people with learning difficulties have also recorded *unedited* versions of their experience. See for example 'Joyce's story' written by Joyce Kershaw (in Goodley 2000: 88–96) and Lewis Smith's (2000b) 'A nebulous state of mind with an euphorious attitude'.

Other people with learning difficulties, either individually or in groups, may welcome opportunities to compile a record of their lived experiences. There are many different ways in which this can be achieved, for example: photograph albums (with or without captions); pictures or artwork; drama productions, videos or audiotapes. Alternatively people can be supported to write their own life stories, or their spoken words can be transcribed. Lewis Smith, who was supported by students from the learning difficulties degree, made a video and an audio tape, both of which were later transcribed and have recently been published (Smith 2000a, b).

Supporting and encouraging people to formulate their own ideas and theories about their experiences

Some people with learning difficulties are formulating their own ideas about their experiences. For example, Art and Power, a group from Bristol, have conceptualised their experience of oppression by the medical profession as doctors *lying* to them (and/or their parents) about their potential. With support, they made a video entitled *The Lying Doctors* which explains, forcefully and powerfully, the reasons why they understand their experience in this way (Art and Power 1998).

In order to formulate their ideas, people with learning difficulties may need support from other people with learning difficulties, so that ideas can be developed *collectively*. They may also need help from advisers or supporters without learning difficulties. It may also be helpful for people with learning difficulties to have access to other people's research, ideas and theories about their lives and experiences.

Sharing research findings about people with learning difficulties

Some summaries of research findings are being produced which are more accessible to people with learning difficulties. For example, The Norah Fry Research Centre at the University of Bristol has produced a series of accessible summaries entitled *Plain Facts* (Townsley 1998). It is also possible for supporters to talk through or 'translate' other research findings in order to make them more accessible. The findings and conclusions of some studies, however, may be very negative (for example, McConnell and Llwellyn 2000) and supporters may find it difficult to share these. People with learning difficulties may, however, be only too aware of discrimination and may have frequent experience of being subjected to other people's negative ideas about their potential. They may also have some awareness of wider issues through television programmes covering disability and learning difficulties (see Chapter 10). Dan Goodley (2000: 3) refers to people with learning difficulties' 'resilience in the face of adversity'. This resilience should perhaps be borne in mind when making decisions about facilitating their access to negative information.

Explaining theories and ideas about people with learning difficulties

If people with learning difficulties are to be included in debate that theorises their lives and experiences, they may wish to have opportunities to find out about other people's theoretical ideas. Some theorising about the social model and people with learning difficulties is complex (for example, Dowse 2001; Goodley 2001). The basic idea of the social model is, however, fairly straightforward, as I have tried to indicate above. Some people with learning difficulties, with support, can gain an understanding of the basic principles of the social model of disability and may conceptualise their oppression as disabled people as *unfair treatment* by services or discriminatory policies. See, for example, Michaela Jones and Shaun Smith's comments in Chapter 10.

Offering support to people with additional needs

People with learning difficulties who also have sensory impairments or communication difficulties may need additional support in order to document their experiences or contribute to discussion. People with learning difficulties who also experience mental and emotional distress or challenging behaviours may also wish to participate and consideration would need to be given to their support needs.

Offering emotional support

There is evidence that some of the people with learning difficulties who were institutionalised during the twentieth century were subjected to brutality and abuse (Martin 1984; Potts and Fido 1991; Barron 1996). There is also more recent evidence of abuse in community-based services (Harris and Craft 1994; Roeher Institute 1995). It is possible that people with learning difficulties who wish to document or theorise their experience may themselves have been abused. It is imperative therefore that support is made available if people become distressed. One important form of support is that of other people with learning difficulties who have lived through similar distressing experiences.

Respecting people's views about sharing their experiences and publication

Some people with learning difficulties may welcome support to record their experiences but may prefer not to share or publicise their work. Others (for example, Barron 1996; Smith 2000a, b) want as many people as possible to know about their experiences. It is important that people's views are respected and efforts made to minimise the risk of people being 'persuaded' to publish experiences they would prefer to keep private.

Clearly, it won't be possible to involve every person with learning difficulties in recording or theorising their experiences. Some people may have little or no interest in becoming involved. Others would need extensive support in order to participate; such support may, or may not, be available. If some people with learning difficulties are involved in theorising their experiences, it is likely that the 'representativeness' of those people will be questioned (Beresford and Campbell 1994). Such involvement would, however, be congruent with the disabled people's movement which *challenges*:

> traditional views of disabled people as incapable, powerless and passive and in so-doing, establishes disabled people and their organisations as the 'experts' on disability and disability related issues.
>
> (Oliver and Barnes 1998: 71)

The alternative – other people (without learning difficulties) theorising *on behalf of* people with learning difficulties – appears to be more in keeping with traditional (individual model) views of people with learning difficulties as 'incapable, powerless and passive'.

A unifying social model of disability

Colin Barnes (1998) argues that literature produced by critics of the social model of disability which focuses on the pain, fatigue and depression of impairment is similar to literature produced by medical sociologists. Such literature reinforces negative stereotypes of disabled people and detracts attention away from the disabling environments and wider social structures highlighted by social model approaches. By reducing the collective institutional discrimination and oppression of disability to the personal tragedy and 'individual deficit' of impairment, the social model critics' focus on impairment also 'effectively blurs the distinction between experience of impairment and experience of disability' (Barnes 1998: 77).

Within the disabled people's movement, a number of authors have counselled against focusing upon personal experiences of impairment (for example, Hunt 1998 [1966]; Oliver 1996a; Barnes 1998) because of concerns about replicating individual model approaches. Contrary to this, as Jan Walmsley (2001) points out, in relation to people with learning difficulties, much of the inclusive research being undertaken is focused upon people with learning difficulties' personal experiences. This takes the form of 'narrative style research, based on biography, life history, oral history or accounts of personal experience of services' (Walmsley 2001: 199). Indeed, some of the suggestions I outline above for including people with learning difficulties in social model discussion could also be viewed as falling into this category. I would, however, still wish to actively support and promote such approaches. There are two important reasons for this.

The first is that the involvement of people with learning difficulties in social model discussion is relatively new. In the early days of the development of the social model of disability, there was considerable discussion of individual disabled people's experiences of both impairment and disability. It was through the sharing of these individual experiences that people became aware of their collective experience of disability (Campbell and Oliver 1996; Barnes 1998; Oliver and Barnes 1998). Individual experiences of disability continue to be included in social model discussion; for example, Michael Oliver (1996b), a key proponent of the social model, includes a retrospective account of his personal experiences in one of his more recent books.

The second reason is that defenders of the social model are concerned about social model critics' focus on personal experiences of *impairment* (rather than personal experiences of *disability*). Dan Goodley's 'inclusive' social model of disability points to the socially constructed nature of people with learning difficulties' 'impairments':

> The 'difference' of people with learning difficulties, understood as being located in some biological deficit, individualizes their very humanity: ripping them out of a social context, placing them in the realms of pathological curiosity . . . the social model of disability can only include people with learning difficulties when it recognizes the social origins of 'learning difficulties' and 'difference'.
>
> (Goodley 2000: 35)

In Goodley's 'inclusive' social model, therefore, discussion of people with learning difficulties' experiences of 'impairment' will be discussion of the 'social origins of "learning difficulties" and "difference"' or, in social model terms, discussion of their experiences of '*disability*'.

Within the broader disabled people's movement, critics of the social model have also pointed to the marginalisation of the experiences of Black disabled people and other minority groups (for example, Vernon 1998). It may be that people with learning difficulties' experience has more in common with these discussions than discussions of the pain, fatigue and depression of impairment. Ayesha Vernon suggests that despite differences in the experiences of people from minority groups:

> there is one critical similarity in the experience of all disabled people *arising from the stigma of impairment* which often overrides all other boundaries of 'race', gender, sexuality, class and age.
>
> (Vernon 1998: 208, emphasis added)

Irrespective of whether that impairment is considered a biologically based 'individual deficit' or a socially constructed '*perceived* impairment' (Barnes 1998: 78), people with learning difficulties also experience the *stigma of impairment*. This commonality of experience with other disabled people provides a unifying force for the inclusion of people with learning difficulties within the social model of disability.

If people with learning difficulties are to share in the progress and developments of the disabled people's movement, it is important that discussions of their inclusion within the social model of disability highlight commonality, rather than 'difference'.

References

Art and Power (1998) *The Lying Doctors*, Bristol, Community Arts Project Ltd.

Aspis, S. (1999) What they don't tell disabled people with learning difficulties. In: M. Corker and S. French, *Disability Discourse*, Buckingham, Open University Press, pp 173–182.

Atkinson, D. and Williams, F. (eds) (1990) *'Know Me As I Am': An Anthology of Prose, Poetry and Art by People with Learning Difficulties*, London, Hodder & Stoughton.

Atkinson, D., Jackson, M. and Walmsley, J. (eds) (1997) *Forgotten Lives: Exploring the History of Learning Disability*, Plymouth, BILD.

Barnes, C. (1991) *Disabled People in Britain and Discrimination: A Case for Anti-discrimination Legislation*, London, Hurst & Company.

Barnes, C. (1998) The social model of disability: a sociological phenomenon ignored by sociologists?'. In: T. Shakespeare (ed.) *The Disability Reader: Social Sciences Perspectives*, London, Cassell, pp 65–78.

Barnes, C., Mercer, G. and Shakespeare, T. (1999) *Exploring Disability: A Sociological Introduction*, Cambridge, Polity Press.

Baron, S., Riddell, R. and Wilkinson, H. (1998) The best burgers? The person with learning difficulties as worker. In: T. Shakespeare (ed.) *The Disability Reader: Social Sciences Perspectives*, London, Cassell, pp 94–109.

Barron, D. (1996) *A Price to Be Born: My Childhood and Life in a Mental Institution*, Harrogate, Mencap Northern Division.

Barron, D. (2001) Lecture to BA (Hons) Professional Studies: Learning Difficulties students, Stockport College, 10 January.

Beresford, P. and Campbell, J. (1994) Disabled people, services users, user involvement and representation, *Disability & Society*, 9(3): 315–325.

Branfield, F. (1998) What are you doing here? 'Non-disabled' people and the disability movement: a response to Robert F. Drake, *Disability & Society*, 13(1): 143–144.

Branfield, F. (2000) Book review: Jenkins, R. (ed.) (1998) *Questions of Competence: Culture, Classification and Intellectual Disability*, *Disability & Society*, 15(2): 371–374.

Brisenden, S. (1998 [1986]) Independent living and the medical model of disability. In: T. Shakespeare (ed.) *The Disability Reader: Social Sciences Perspectives*, London, Cassell, pp 20–27.

Campbell, J. and Oliver, M. (1996) *Disability Politics: Understanding our Past, Changing our Future*, London, Routledge.

Chappell, A.L. (1998) Still out in the cold, people with learning difficulties and the social model of disability. In: T. Shakespeare (ed.) *The Disability Reader*, London, Cassell, pp 211–220.

Chappell, A.L., Goodley, D. and Lawthom, R. (2001) Making connections: the relevance of the social model of disability for people with learning difficulties, *British Journal of Learning Disabilities*, 29(2): 45–50.

Crow, L. (1996) Including all of our lives: renewing the social model of disability. In: J. Morris (ed.) *Encounters with Strangers: Feminism and Disability*, London, The Women's Press.

Davis, L. (ed.) (1997) *The Disability Studies Reader*, London, Routledge.

Department of Health (2001) *Valuing People: A New Strategy for Learning Disability for the 21st Century*, London, The Stationery Office.

Dowse, L. (2001) Contesting practices, challenging codes: self advocacy, disability politics and the social model, *Disability & Society*, 16(1): 123–141.

Finkelstein, V. (1981) 'To deny or not to deny disability. In: A. Brechin, P. Liddiard and J. Swain (eds) *Handicap in a Social World*, Sevenoaks, Hodder & Stoughton, pp 34–36.

French, S. (1993) Disability, impairment or something in between? In: J. Swain, V. Finkelstein, S. French and M. Oliver (eds) *Disabling Barriers – Enabling Environments*, London, Sage.

Goodley, D. (2000) *Self-advocacy in the Lives of People with Learning Difficulties*, Buckingham, Open University Press.

Goodley, D. (2001) 'Learning difficulties', the social model of disability and impairment: challenging epistemologies, *Disability & Society*, 16(2): 207–223.

Harris, J. and Craft, A. (eds) (1994) *People with Learning Disabilities at Risk of Physical or Sexual Abuse*, BILD Seminar Paper No 4, Kidderminster, BILD.

Hunt, N. (1967) *The World of Nigel Hunt*, Beaconsfield, Darwen Finlayson.

Hunt, P. (1998 [1966]) A critical condition. In: T. Shakespeare (ed.) *The Disability Reader: Social Sciences Perspectives*, London, Cassell.

Lakin, D. (2000) My daughter Melanie. In: P. Murray and J. Penman (eds) *Telling Our Own Stories: Reflections on Family Life in a Disabling World*, Sheffield, Parents with Attitude, pp 43–49.

MacMahon, J. (1955) *Minutes of Evidence of the Royal Commission on the Law Relating to Mental Illness and Mental Deficiency, 30th day*, HMSO, London.

Marks, D. (1999) *Disability: Controversial Debates and Psychosocial Perspectives*, London, Routledge.

Martin, J. (1984) *Hospitals in Trouble*, Oxford, Blackwell.

McConnell, D. and Llwellyn, G. (2000) Disability and discrimination in statutory child protection proceedings, *Disability & Society*, 15(6): 883–895.

Morris, J. (1991) *Pride Against Prejudice: Transforming Attitudes to Disability*, London, The Women's Press.

Morris, J. (1993) *Independent Lives: Community Care and Disabled People*, Basingstoke, Macmillan.

Morris, J. (1996) (ed.) *Encounters with Strangers: Feminism and Disability*, London, The Women's Press.

Murray, P. and Penman, J. (1996) *Let Our Children Be: A Collection of Stories*, Sheffield, Parents with Attitude.

Murray, P. and Penman, J. (eds) (2000) *Telling Our Own Stories: Reflections on Family Life in a Disabling World*, Sheffield, Parents with Attitude.

O'Connor, N. and Tizard, J. (1956) *The Social Problem of Mental Deficiency*, London, Pergamon Press.

Oliver, M. (1990) *The Politics of Disablement*, Basingstoke, Macmillan.

Oliver, M. (1996a) Defining impairment and disability: issues at stake. In: C. Barnes and G. Mercer (eds) *Exploring the Divide: Illness and Disability*, Leeds, The Disability Press.

Oliver, M. (1996b) *Understanding Disability: from Theory to Practice*, Basingstoke, Macmillan.

Oliver, M. and Barnes, C. (1998) *Social Policy and Disabled People: From Exclusion to Inclusion*, London, Longman.

Potts, M. and Fido, R. (1991) *'A Fit Person to be Removed': Personal Accounts of Life Within a Mental Deficiency Institution*, Plymouth, Northcote House.

Roeher Institute (1995) *Harm's Way: The Many Faces of Violence and Abuse Against Persons with Disabilities*, North York, Roeher Institute.

Ryan, J.and Thomas, F. (1987) *The Politics of Mental Handicap*, London, Free Association Books.

Smith, L. (2000a) 'Lewis'. In: P. Murray and J. Penman (eds) *Telling Our Own Stories: Reflections on Family Life in a Disabling World*, Sheffield, Parents with Attitude, pp 17–19.

Smith, L. (2000b) A nebulous state of mind with an euphorious attitude. In: P. Murray and J. Penman (eds) *Telling Our Own Stories: Reflections on Family Life in a Disabling World*, Sheffield, Parents with Attitude, pp 20–27.

Sutcliffe, J. and Simons, K. (1993) *Self-advocacy and Adults with Learning Difficulties: Contexts and Debates*, Leicester, National Institute of Adult Continuing Education.

Thomson, M. (1998) *The Problem of Mental Deficiency: Eugenics, Democracy, and Social Policy in Britain c.1870–1959*, Oxford, Clarendon Press.

Tomlinson, S. (1982) *A Sociology of Special Education*, London, Routledge & Kegan Paul.

Townsley, R. (1998) Information is power: The impact of accessible information on people with learning difficulties. In: L. Ward (ed.) *Innovations in Advocacy and Empowerment for People with Intellectual Disabilities*, Chorley, Lisieux Hall Publications.

Vernon, A. (1998) 'Multiple oppression and the Disabled People's Movement. In: T. Shakespeare (ed.) *The Disability Reader: Social Sciences Perspectives*, London, Cassell, pp 201–210.

Vonnegut, K. (1969) Harrison Bergeron. In: K. Vonnegut (ed.) *Welcome to the Monkey House*, London, Jonathan Cape, pp 7–13.

Walmsley, J. (2001) Normalisation, emancipatory research and inclusive research in learning disability, *Disability & Society*, 16(2): 187–205.

Wilding, P. (1982) *Professional Power and Social Welfare*, London, Routledge & Kegan Paul.

Williams, P. (1999) Hearing the voice of people with Down's Syndrome, *Community Living*, 12(4): 10–11.

Chapter 13

Conclusion – a personal reflection on values, learning disability and a social approach

David Race

Introduction

This final chapter attempts to pull together, by way of a personal reflection, the underlying themes of this book. As I noted in the Introduction, adopting a social approach to both a degree course and a textbook revealed the tensions between the expectations and demands of the academic world and the paths down which the social approach would tend to lead us as teachers and writers. The result is, I hope and believe, that the tension has been used creatively, and that those who have read thus far have a sense of how learning disability services, the theoretical and policy arguments that surround them, and the real lives of those who use them are also a precarious balance of those tensions.

This final reflection will use three stories to try and summarise those tensions, and to put the case that any attempts to work creatively and radically in this field will very quickly bring one to a point of decision about values. What one then goes on to do will depend to a large extent on those values, including, if one is attempting to teach and write about learning disability, how one does that, and what gets communicated.

The conclusion that some readers may draw from the various chapters in this book might well be a somewhat negative one, regarding the way people are treated, and the lives they have led. This would not be without foundation, as again I noted in the Introduction, and looking at the number of times those with some length of time in the field have used the phrase *plus ça change*. Equally, however, it is to be hoped that some of the developments noted throughout the book, in ways of involving people, in the opportunities created by the *Valuing People* White Paper (though these must be taken up locally if they are to bear fruit), give readers some sense that things can be achieved, and that there is worthwhile work to do. The scale of that work, however, and the examination of values necessary to undertake it, is what this final chapter will attempt to illustrate.

Challenging human services – lessons from a module

As we told the students on the degree course at the start of the module with the same title as this section, this particular series of sessions was the hardest to describe and yet, from feedback, the one from which the students drew the most. Since it also evolved in response to their feedback, in terms of the emphasis on its various components, it is not surprising perhaps that it was greeted with the degree of effort and honest reflection that it was. The content dwelt on a number of issues that have already been covered in this book, in particular the 'normalisation debate' (see Chapter 11), issues of 'corruption of care' with regard to how people had been and were treated in services (see various chapters), and the ethical issues surrounding pre-natal screening and selective abortion of impaired children. A lot of the teaching involved the sharing of experiences, and it was initially surprising, and then expected, as each year group's experience was confirmed by the following one, how consistent and widespread were the parallels that students drew from their own jobs or placements in learning disability services with the issues we as teachers were raising.

One exercise especially illustrates my point in this section. Students were asked to think about incidents in their service experience (many of our students had or were working in services, and all students had two practical placements) under two headings. One, where something happened and they would have liked to challenge, but didn't, and one where they did challenge what was going on. We ourselves (the course was taught by Kathy Boxall and myself) told our own incidents addressing the same points, and this usually freed students from some initial anxiety about talking about situations where they might have been seen to have acted cautiously, or even, as some of them put it, 'been too scared'.

The overwhelming result of these discussions, in direct parallel with analyses of the 'hospital scandals' of the 1960s and 1970s, or much more recent incidents, such as those uncovered by a 'Face the Facts' radio programme, were as follows. First, the number of incidents where people thought they should have challenged practice in some way but did not far outweighed the number of incidents where they did. Second, even where some challenge to a situation was made, it was rarely resolved either in favour of the people with learning difficulties, or even without some retribution on the person doing the challenging. Third, the power of 'custom and practice', organisational survival, and personal power politics within services invariably won the day over 'idealistic' arguments about valuing people, or issues of dignity and rights.

This, again, should not surprise those who have read this book, or indeed those who have worked for any length of time in human services. What, for me, was more worrying was that the discussions over values issues, which had certainly been to the fore in the first two decades of my involvement with learning disability services, now seemed to be confined to the classroom situation, and even there a number of students were reluctant to get into the dangerous territory that values debate can be.

So we seem to be in the essentially postmodern position of all having values, but, like Victorians and sex, it doesn't make for polite conversation. The difficulty for our subject, I believe, is that people with learning difficulties bring values into sharp focus, with both the dark side of our human nature and its opposite being roused by their vulnerability. To work in services day after day often means those values are repressed into unconsciousness, either to avoid facing unpleasant realities or, more often, simply to get on with the work that needs to be done. Simply to reduce work with people to a set of tasks, however, can never, in my view, eradicate the values issues, but merely squeeze them into one corner of our lives, only for them to reappear, like the other edge of a squeezed balloon, somewhere else. This segmentation of thinking about issues is illustrated by the next story.

The midwives tale – compartmentalising lives

As this book was being written I attended an informal internal seminar at the university at which I work. The speaker was talking about research for her higher degree dissertation that had involved carrying out a series of open-ended interviews with midwives who were giving advice about pre-natal screening and selective abortion of babies with Down's syndrome. The trigger for the research had been her own experience in having to give advice about 'test results' that suggested a probability of Down's syndrome, leading to a decision by the mother whether to have a full amniocentesis and, if Down's syndrome were established, a termination. This is now commonplace, but at the point only five or so years ago when the researcher, in her job as a midwife, was asked to give this advice, it was not done uniformly. In fact in her region of the city these tests were not carried out, but some mothers who lived in her administrative 'patch' happened to have a maternity hospital from another area that was more convenient for them to attend, and this hospital was promoting these tests. So our researching midwife, who had at that point heard little about the tests, let alone had any formal training on the subject, was expected to go and 'advise' women who had, in the telling phrase, a 'bad result'.

Given that experience, she then decided to find out the views of midwives on this process, and their part in it. Since she may well be publishing her results, I do not intend to go into them here, but to draw from them two issues and one anecdote connected to my overall theme. The first issue is how unconnected midwives felt to the momentum of the process. It was as if the assumption was already made that having a child with Down's syndrome was automatically bad, and that as midwives, it was their duty to put that over to the mothers. Those who had adopted a broader counselling approach, sometimes with the result that mothers did not want to proceed with testing, found themselves overruled by doctors the next time the mothers visited the hospital.

The second issue was how no account seemed to be taken of the values position of the midwives. While there still seems to be a 'conscience clause' for nurses who do not want to work in abortion services, those midwives who either felt strongly about abortion as such or about abortion of disabled children did not appear to have such an option. Indeed, in general discussion at the seminar, it appears that a 'battery of tests' are now offered to women as routine procedure, with only those with the knowledge and values position to definitely opt out being able to refuse them. As with our students in their work places, it seemed to me that the midwives were being expected to segment their values between work and outside, and to suppress any challenge to the prevailing view of Down's syndrome. Interestingly, when I raised a question as to whether midwives in training ever met anyone with Down's syndrome, I was told, by older midwives in the audience that 'we used to have a session on it but they don't any more'. Even that 'session' had been a lecture by an 'expert' rather than actually getting to meet somebody with Down's syndrome.

The anecdote told by the researcher concerned a story by one of her interviewees that makes the segmenting point still further. The interviewee midwife had just had a particularly long session with a mother who had had a 'bad result' culminating in that mother opting for an amniocentesis and possible termination. On her way home the midwife was accustomed to pick up her young daughter from primary school, and go home with her on the bus. As they travelled on this particular day, another mother and her daughter got on the bus, as it stopped by a different school. The little girl had Down's syndrome, and, as children will, the midwife's little girl asked, not 'what is wrong with that little girl?' but 'why does that little girl look different?'. The contrast, in trying to explain to her own daughter about Down's syndrome with the somewhat formulaic 'advice' that she had given the mother that day was not lost on the interviewee. As she said, as best as I can recall the story, 'It made me really think – what are we doing? Who's to say that there shouldn't be people with Down's syndrome?'

A village story – fear and prejudice at the turn of the millennium

The last story is the longest, but readers are asked for their forbearance as I think it summarises the themes of this book, even down to the use of language and terminology. It is a true story, though names and locations have been changed in this account to conceal identification of those who have not given permission for their names to be used. The principal character has asked for the story to be told.

Mary is a university lecturer. She lives, as she has done for the past twenty-five years, in a small village of some 350 people in a rural area in the south of England some thirty miles from the city where she works. Mary's specialism is learning disability, and as well as teaching on a course not unlike the one described in this book she has a personal interest in the subject. With her partner Alan, who works for the Social Services Department of a different city, she has raised four sons, who in 1999, when the main events of this story took place, were aged 14, 16, 19 and 20. The youngest of these, Joshua, had been adopted at the age of 6 months. Joshua has Down's syndrome, and Mary used to tell the following story about him to illustrate the values issues in learning disability. He had been born, she would relate, in a market town on the other side of the county. Had he been born some ten miles further north, in a city in the next county, there was a high probability that he would still have been with his natural parents. That city's Social Services Department had a reconciliation scheme that had a 90 per cent success rate in re-uniting parents and disabled children who had initially been rejected. Had Joshua been conceived some twenty miles further south, in yet a third county and its major city, there was an equally high chance that he would not have been born at all. That city's university hospital was pioneering much wider use of amniocentesis than was then common, and had thus been doing a wider 'sweep' of mothers. Had Joshua's mother lived in that city there was a high chance she would have been selected for a test, and thus a high chance that he would have been aborted. As it was, the sleepy market town maternity hospital where he was born simply responded to the rejection of Joshua by his parents by placing him for adoption, some twenty-four hours after his birth.

Hence his adoption by Mary and Alan. As they raised Joshua and his three brothers in the village he was welcomed by people in their own quiet way. Babysitters and childminders who had taken the elder boys showed a willingness to take Joshua, and some surprise when he was not really very different to deal with. The local nursery school took all the boys, as did, after some dispute with the county who wanted to put him in a 'special unit', the village school, which served as an infant school before children went to junior schools in the nearest town. Mary, in fact, used to say that Joshua had 'taught the village a lot' by his presence. The only previous contact with learning disability had been two other people with Down's syndrome in earlier decades, both of whom had left the village by 1999.

As mentioned, Joshua attended the village school at the infant age, 5 to 7, before going on to the town junior school. The head who had been concerned about his coming to the village school (which was at that point an annexe of the town school) was in the process of changing into an ardent advocate of inclusive education, at least as far as Joshua was concerned. The head and governors were also, however, with pressure from the Local Authority Education Department, seeking to close the village school, and this was eventually done, like many others in the Thatcher era, in the name of 'value for money'. Some complicated legal searching eventually established that the school building was owned by the local diocese of the Church of England and they proposed to sell it as a possible conversion to residential property. As well as the school closure, the 1980s and early 1990s, again like many rural villages elsewhere, brought many new people to the village, converting barns and other buildings, even the Methodist chapel, into residential property. The few council houses that there had been were mostly sold off to their sitting tenants, the number of three-generation families and the number of farms diminished, and the number of holiday cottages increased.

This brings us back to 1999, when the main events of this story unfolded. For the previous ten years Mary had been Chair of the committee of the village hall, a large, two-storey building, constructed after the First World War, and once boasting the finest dance floor in that part of the county. The committee had been formed in the late 1980s when, in response to a desperate appeal from the trustees, descendants of the original village worthies who had built the place, the trust had been turned into a charity, owned by the whole village. The desperate call had come because the building was falling into severe disrepair due to lack of use, and public meetings to try and do something about it had had single-figure attendance. Over the ten years that followed, after basic repairs had kept the building going, the brief flurry of interest that surrounded the change to charity status had subsided to the previous state of apathy. At the annual meeting in late 1998, the attendance was seven, all of whom were committee members, and of those a number were looking to resign. For most of these ten years, the school building had been in limbo, while ownership was established, and a response from the village awaited as to whether there might be a 'community use' for the building, which the diocese had requested.

So the new committee elected at that meeting in 1998 determined to attempt something they had investigated earlier, only for their plans to be thwarted due to lack of support from the district council. This was to sell the village hall, and replace it with a conversion to the school building, which was in much better repair. To do this, under the terms of the charity, they needed to call a meeting of the whole village, and obtain a 75 per cent majority in favour. The meeting was called, and attended by about fifty people, something of a record for such meetings. After a full discussion, a vote was taken, and the majority obtained. The committee then employed a local surveyor and estate agent to cost out the repairs to the school and to put the village hall on the market. The price it was valued at would be enough to buy the school and do it up, and negotiations at that end were well under way.

Meanwhile the hall was put on the market, with a guide price set at the level given by the agent. A few enquiries were made, and some offers below the set price, but the committee were advised to wait, as the balance of money was tight. While this was happening Mary went for a walk with a student. This was John, a mature student on Mary's course, who was in his final year. During his second year placement, Anne, one of the people with whom John worked, liked to go for country walks. As part of her placement supervision of John, Mary had joined in one or two of these walks, and they had become a biannual event after the placement finished. So John, Anne and Mary went for a walk in the country, not far from Mary's village, in April of 1999, just after the village hall had gone up for sale. As they walked by a river they came across an old derelict mill being renovated for holiday flats, with a 'For Sale' sign attached. Mary remarked, in general conversation, that the village hall was for sale, and they walked on, talking of other things.

The following week the agent called Mary, asking her to call a committee meeting, since they had received an offer above the asking price, and he thought they should accept. It turned out that the offer was from John and his wife. They wanted to convert the hall into a house for themselves, their two teenage children, and to have two rooms set aside for what was then called 'respite care' for people with learning difficulties. The meeting was held, and the committee voted unanimously to accept the offer. All then seemed to be proceeding well. The groups who used the hall were involved in the plans for the village school conversion, price negotiations were begun with the diocese, and John and his wife visited the hall, and had pleasant conversations with the few people who were there at the time. At that point Mary, Alan and two of the boys went on holiday for three weeks.

The day after their return, in mid-July, a committee member was knocking on the door. He proceeded to tell them of a meeting that had been called by the parish council, where John and his wife had offered to meet people in the village. This had been in response to the formal notice that planning permission was being sought to convert the hall to 'residential use'. The few people who had been opposed all along to the hall being sold, most of whom lived next door or opposite, had exercised their right to see the plans and, though it was not necessary for the planning process, had discovered that John and his family were to offer two of their rooms for respite care. The meeting that then ensued was extremely traumatic for John and his wife. They were almost abused, and faced an extremely hostile audience convinced that the hall was going to be turned into a 'hostel' for all sorts of social services clients, who would then attract drug addicts and 'other undesirables'. John, who was very quietly spoken, had a job to make himself heard, and when he used the term that he had been taught at university to use – 'learning difficulties' – the audience did not know what he was talking about. Though a few villagers spoke in their favour, John and his wife left the meeting in deep depression, and contemplated withdrawing their offer there and then. Since the planning application was still going through, however, and since their offer was still the one accepted by the committee, they decided to continue.

On the same day as the worried committee member visited, Mary had a phone call from one of the leaders of the 'opposition' telling her that feelings were running high and what was she going to do about it. She replied that a meeting of the committee had been set up, and that if anyone wanted to reconsider the sale in the light of the concerns then they could discuss and vote on it. She also prepared a draft of a letter to all the villagers, explaining the committee's decision, and also telling them the legal position, which was that, as a charity, the committee were under an obligation to sell to the highest offer. In the few days that followed, the 'opponent', having interpreted Mary's remarks as meaning that the committee were going to make a final decision, had organised a petition, which stated that the committee were proposing to sell the hall as a 'respite care hostel'. Mary and the committee were then met as they tried to enter the village hall by what can only be described as a mob, of twenty or so people, shouting abuse and demanding that they attend the committee meeting, and that the petition should be the reason to vote to reject John's offer. The degree of hostility was directed primarily at Mary, since rumours had been spreading since the public meeting. These included: that she had set the whole thing up to let her 'friends' get the hall cheap; that those 'friends' had a string of 'respite homes' around the county; that the agent was in on the deal, and had been from the beginning; and so on. Ironically, as Chair, Mary had not voted in any of the decisions, which had all been unanimous. She eventually got into the meeting. In fact, the committee did not have any proposition to alter the sale of the hall. They endorsed Mary's letter explaining the sale and agreed to include a deadline for any other bids to be received, since they were still legally obliged to accept the highest offer. Running the gauntlet of the crowd outside, which had now grown as these things do, and which now included physical threats to the agent, Mary told them to read the letter, and then if they wanted to call a public meeting, they were within their rights to do so.

For the next two weeks, the 'opposition' spread their attack, via letters to villagers, and now turned their campaign from a 'stop the hostel' into a 'save the village hall.' Eventually, as the deadline for any higher bids was approaching, without any being received, the Chair of the Parish Council called a public meeting on the issue. Again, about fifty people attended the meeting, including Mary, Alan, and their two elder sons, who as adults were entitled to vote. Afterwards Mary likened it to a public pillorying, though when the adrenalin died down she acknowledged that it had also revealed a few people from the village who had the courage to stand up for people with learning difficulties. In the main, though, despite explanations of the legal position from Alan, who tried to explain that the home would have to be registered, that it would be inspected, and that no other groups of service users could be housed there, people had not come for a debate, but an execution. Mary tried to explain that anyone could buy any of the vacant properties in the village and, provided that they satisfied the inspection criteria, could have two people for respite care. She also tried to explain the term 'learning difficulties', as did Joshua's brothers by reference to Joshua himself. But in the end Mary was left to reflect that, for all her degrees, publications and acting out of a value position on learning disability by adopting Joshua, the truth that she taught about societal attitudes had come home to roost. One of the committee described it as being 'like racism' and described herself as being physically scared by the hatred on people's faces. People who did not attend also spoke of being too frightened to do so. All the dark side of human nature which I noted at the start of this conclusion was there – fear of the unknown, political jealousy, even the class divisions which usually are much less evident in a village, and all, as Mary said in a resigned statement at the end, for two unknown people with learning difficulties.

The meeting voted, in an almost total reverse of the March meeting, to stop the whole process of selling the hall and buying the school. Mary and the committee resigned en masse, and their places were taken by the leaders of the 'opposition'. Scars were created between villagers that, even two years later, have still to heal. The new committee, bigger in number than the whole annual meeting of the year before, tried to revive the hall, got some grants for minor repairs, but are now complaining of the apathy of the village in not using the hall. The village school remains unsold, though now with planning permission for change to residential use. John left his job in learning disability services, after being off sick for six months after this affair with stress.

Final thoughts

The values issues raised by that story and this book are as broad as society itself. It has been, and is still for some people, tempting to take learning disability out of society, and simply treat working with people as a set of tasks, to be done by 'trained professionals'. In adopting a 'social approach' to our course and our book we expose ourselves to the society that we have got, not the one we might like to have. We would ask that readers reflect on what it really means to value people for being, not for being something, as they consider what the various authors have written.

If, after that reflection, they are strengthened to meet the challenges that working in this field provides, then this book will have been worthwhile.

Index